Normalities and Abnormalities in Human Movement

Medicine and Sport Science

Founder and Editor from 1969 to 1984
E. Jokl, Lexington, Ky.

Vol. 29

Series Editors
M. Hebbelinck, Brussels
R.J. Shephard, Toronto

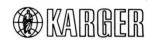

Basel · München · Paris · London · New York · New Delhi · Singapore · Tokyo · Sydney

Normalities and Abnormalities in Human Movement

Volume Editor
B. Kirkcaldy, Düsseldorf

13 figures and 14 tables, 1989

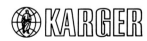

KARGER

Basel · München · Paris · London · New York · New Delhi · Singapore · Tokyo · Sydney

Medicine and Sport Science

Published on behalf of the Research Committee of the International Council of Sport Sciences and Physical Education

Drug Dosage
The authors and the publisher have exerted every effort to ensure that drug selection and dosage set forth in this text are in accord with current recommendations and practice at the time of publication. However, in view of ongoing research, changes in government regulations, and the constant flow of information relating to drug therapy and drug reactions, the reader is urged to check the package insert for each drug for any change in indications and dosage and for added warnings and precautions. This is particularly important when the recommended agent is a new and/or infrequently employed drug.

Dedication

This book is dedicated to two women who have influenced me –

Elizabeth, and
Lisenka, my daughter

In addition, it is intended as a note of gratitude to

Dieter Vaitl, Professor of Psychology,
University of Giessen

Contents

Preface

There are plenty of books that have been written about movement and motor skills, perception and action, psychology and sport, motor skills acquisition, motor development, etc., but few have directed their attention towards the issue of movement behaviour as a psychodiagnostic and therapeutic medium. And those few that have attempted such an exercise, have generally relied on outdated studies involving a low quality of research, and atheoretical inquiry. Since there is no definitive book in this area, the primary aim of this 'reference' book was to provide a 'coherent package', blending therapeutic interventions with differential motodiagnostics.

It further seeks to fill the gap between theoretical concepts from the differential psychomotoric domain and practical applications of methods of movement analysis: Some of the central themes dealt with, include the extent and manner to which movement behaviour can be used as a diagnostic instrument, to determine for example, the development of motor processes in infants and children, psychological disturbances made visible through movement, and the influence of negative emotional states on movement. The unified approach offers a compact set of contemporary reviews fulfilling the requirements of a wide group of interested professions such as rehabilitation counsellors, somatotherapists, psychotherapists and clinical psychologists, physical educators, psychomotor therapists, and kinesiotherapists. The proposals for explorative future research and extensive bibliography will ensure its popularity not only amongst professionals working in the field of human movement, but as a supplementary text for researchers and graduates also.

The interdisciplinary perspective throughout is transparent in the subdivision of the chapters: The book is roughly divided up into two sections, the first intended to deal primarily with diagnostic aspects of movement, and the second, therapeutic aspects. In addition, an attempt has been made to incorporate chapters which encompassed normalities and abnormalities in movement and motor skills. The distinction was felt to be a useful one since there appears to be a progressively developing gap between clinical aspects of motor behaviour and normal functioning in motor skills (Heuer, 1988). It is clear that the sections are not all-embracing and what is more, deal with overlapping topics. Nevertheless, this approximate classification provided a useful guide in the structuring of the book.

The opening chapter, 'Motor behavior, personality and mental abnormality' by Steven Vandenberg begins with an examination of motor behaviour and its measurement in adults and children. A discussion follows of attempts to arrive at motor performance factors, e.g. Oseretsky and Fleischman (psychomotor and physical proficiency factors), including definitions and measures of physical performance components, an examination of Berger's work relating body size with athletic performance, and models of physical performance. The interrelationship between these measures and normal variation in personality is explored, introducing such trait constructs as proposed by Zuckerman and Eysenck. Several studies are selected from sport psychology aimed at identifying the personality of various athletes. In addition, several sections review investigations from occupational, e.g. Holland's typology of vocational interests, interpersonal behaviour (based on Sullivan's theory), as well as recreational and leisure time activities, e.g. McKenzie's work. Finally, impaired or deviant motor behaviour of mental patients is considered: this includes reference to Yate's analysis of psychomotor deficits amongst mentally ill patients, and aspects of the Luria-Nebraska neuropsychological test. Spontaneous and drug-induced movement disorders are examined, including psychoactive drugs which influence movement, and the effect of body types on expressive style.

The chapter by Herbert Heuer presents a selective and evaluative review of the major hypotheses on mental practice effects. The hypotheses are organized within a multiple-representations framework of skilled movement. In accordance with this framework, different kinds of representations have to be distinguished. Mental practice consists in the manipulation of some of these. The cognitive hypothesis suggests that its effects are limited to spatiotemporal and symbolic representations. This hypothesis is well supported. Its major implication is that mental practice effects are only found for those skills for which translations of spatiotemporal or symbolic representations into actual motor commands are possible. Otherwise changes of spatiotemporal and symbolic representations remain separated from actual performance.

The traditional ideomotor hypothesis appears to be more acceptable if modified to become a programming hypothesis: according to this hypothesis, part of mental practice effects is due to manipulations of motor and/or kinesthetic representations which are more closely linked to actual performance. Support for this hypothesis is weak. The implications of the various representations that mediate mental practice effects for applications in different fields are discussed.

Warren Eaton offers a review of several statistical integrations (meta-analyses) of the empirical literature on sex differences in motor performance tasks and in motor activity level. The magnitude of sex differences is approached using the concept of the effect size, which is the difference between males and females expressed in standard deviation units. So considered, sex differences on motor performance tasks are generally much smaller before puberty than after. Childhood sex differences on many physical size and body composition measures are, however, shown to be comparable in magnitude to well-established sex differences in other domains. Moreover, differences of such magnitude will tend to be accompanied by noticeable disparities in the number of males and females at performance extremes. Childhood sex differences in activity level, size, and body composition should not be discounted as contributors to motor performance outcomes.

Peter Schwenkmezger and Georg Steffgen provide a contemporary review of the area of anxiety and movement. They note that everyday observation and empirical analyses testify to the fact that the acquisition and performance of motor skills are accompanied by a great number of emotional processes. Because movement also contributes to the satisfaction of biological and social motives, negative emotions, such as anxiety, can also result. The effect of anxiety on the quantitative level of motor performance is discussed on the basis of the following theories: cognitive approaches (interference theories of anxiety, Spielberger's theory, the attention hypothesis of anxiety, and modifications of cognitive approaches, e.g. Wine). Empirical results from research on motor skills emanating from each of these theories are described and discussed.

In motor research, there has been a predominance of studies on the effect of anxiety on performance. Much less interest has been directed to analyses of the quality of movements. This is probably due to the methodological problems inherent in such an approach. Several empirical analyses are, however, available and these are summarized. This review is followed by a discussion of the perspectives presented by this kind of experimental approach. The distinction offered in anxiety research, between anxiety and coping with anxiety, is usually made on methodological or didactic grounds, less often for reasons of content. The theories dealing with movement behaviour are also discussed, including person-related styles of coping, situation-related and transactional theories and models. Finally, the authors suggest practical applications of these findings and examine research perspectives.

The contribution by Theo Manschreck reviews the clinical and experimental literature on pathological motor behaviour in schizophrenia. Dramatic motor disturbances such as catalepsy are less common in this disorder, but more subtle features such as stereotypic or repetitive movements and general clumsiness are frequent. These motor abnormalities are not unique to schizophrenia. Basal ganglia disease, brain damage, drug effects and other disorders may be sources for various anomalities, some of which are similar phenomenologically to those reported in schizophrenic disorder. Thus, the classic motor phenomena of schizophrenic disorders (abnormal voluntary movements) are prominent and unexplained features of this baffling illness. Recent research has (1) investigated the kinds and frequencies of these motor disturbances in schizophrenia and other disorders, (2) distinguished them from those more clearly associated with drug treatment, and (3) detected relationships between motor abnormalities and other aspects of schizophrenic psychopathology. The development of quantitative computer- and laboratory-based methods has emerged as an important strategy for extending our knowledge of motor pathology. New evidence points to potentially important connections between these intrinsic abnormal voluntary movements and abnormal involuntary movements, especially tardive dyskinesia.

Harald Wallbott's chapter does not focus on quantitative aspects of movement in psychopathological disorders, that is, reduced eye contact or gesturing in depressives, etc., but instead on features of movement quality, such as duration, circumference, velocity or acceleration of movements. A review is offered of the relevant psychiatric literature, including several phenomenological descriptions on movement quality changes, with particular emphasis on the German 'expression psychology' movement. There then follows an examination of parameters of movement quality, as well as discussion of some appropriate measuring techniques (based on frame-by-frame coordinate measurements of selected points of the body). In the final section, Wallbott reports on his own studies attempting to identify movement quality parameters which best differentiate the motor behaviour of psychiatric patients prior to and after successful treatment. In addition, a detailed analysis is provided of those parameters which guide observers in inferring psychological state. The results imply that some movement quality parameters are valid indicators of psychopathological state, but that observers seem to use other (invalid) parameters in their judgements, resulting in invalid proximal judgements of psychopathological state.

A central issue of the chapter by Susan Lyons and Maureen Pope is the goal of therapy. Verbal comments are a means of grasping client understanding of their problems, but it is unclear whether verbalization of 'understanding' is equivalent to understanding or coping. The significance of experience and sensing and the need to adopt a more phenomenological approach within therapy is argued. Given the potential problem of overreliance on verbalization, movement therapy is suggested as an alternative approach. This is not to deny the importance of other therapeutic practices but to demonstrate the need to consider alternatives. In particular, the work of Laban and his effort shape notation is discussed and the relation between his ideas and those of George Kelly are considered. Movement can be seen as a form of construing within this framework. It is noted that often Kelly's work is manifested by adherence to repertory grid analysis in the same way as Labanotation seems for many to typify the work of Laban.

The article suggests that Laban and Kelly offer, within their philosophical positions, a much richer source of inspiration for therapists, especially those wishing to engage in encouraging clients to demonstrate their agency through movement. Both men were ultimately interested in the possibilities of people making sense of the world within which they lived. Both valued experience and understanding above accumulative fragmentalism of knowledge. For Kelly, the psychotherapist or teacher, in carrying out their facilitative role, would be engaged in a process whereby the clients/learners could recognize their agency and responsibility for the models of the world they had created and in this way the person would not be a victim of biography. Movement as construing and movement analysis may provide a vehicle for a person's reflective understanding and as a mode of communication between therapists/educator and client as an adjunct or an alternative to more traditional verbal therapies.

Bruce Kirkcaldy's chapter entitled 'Exercise as a therapeutic modality' explores contemporary empirical studies aimed at evaluating the therapeutic effectiveness of vigorous physical activity as a method of stress management, for both clinical and nonclinical groups. Several psychological and physiological theoretical models are considered. There then follows a comprehensive review of the literature, based predominantly on studies published during the last five years, to exemplify some of the central methodological and statistical issues which characterize the area. This includes discussion of the social component of sport participation, the adverse effects of exercise, the problem of the dropout or noncomplier, sampling bias and the related issue of expectancy effects, operationalization of exercise, indices of therapeutic outcome and their clinical significance, individual differences in susceptibility to therapeutic intervention, and the 'endorphin connection'. After evaluation of the quality of research, a resume is offered together with an analysis of the implications of these findings.

The final chapter by Adrian Furnham is primarily concerned with social skills theory and research as it relates specifically to motor behaviour. The diverse and diffuse history of social skills theory is reviewed and the different approaches described. Recent developments and problems in the literature dominated by applied clinical and social psychologists are discussed. The second part of the chapter looks at motor, as opposed to affective or cognitive, components of social skills theory and attempts both a review and a classification of this work. Various questions are asked such as what do movements mean, and to what extent are senders and receivers aware of movements and how easy are motor skills to train? Finally current concerns and future interests of social skills theory are reviewed along with suggestions for its application within the area of sport and movement.

It remains for me to wish that readers share our excitement and satisfaction with the end product. I would be delighted if they provide feedback about their opinion of the book's contents and suggestions for additions and improvements for future publications. Finally, I would like to take this opportunity of thanking the publishers, in particular, Mr. Rolf Steinebrunner of Karger Medical Publishers, Basel, for his support leading to the appearance of this volume. I am particularly pleased that the unfolding of this book corresponds to the celebration of the 600th Anniversary of the University of Cologne!

Bruce Kirkcaldy

Diagnostic Aspects: Normal and Abnormal Groups

Kirkcaldy B (ed): Normalities and Abnormalities in Human Movement.
Med Sport Sci. Basel, Karger, 1989, vol 29, pp 1–35

Motor Behavior, Personality, and Mental Abnormality[1]

Steven G. Vandenberg

Institute for Behavioral Genetics, University of Colorado, Boulder, Colo., USA

When first encountering these terms one tends to wonder if there is any relationship between them at all. Glancing in some introductory texts in psychology makes it clear that such relationships, if they are mentioned at all, certainly are not well known. This suggests that the relationships are either not very strong or, perhaps more likely, not obvious because they are complicated and obscured by other variables: age, sex, socioeconomic status, and body type readily come to mind. In what follows, an attempt will be made to survey briefly what is known and to speculate about possible directions in which to search for more information.

What we are interested in lies in an area bordered by physical education, neurology, psychiatry, kinesiology and sport psychology, leisure time studies, sociology, and cultural anthropology.

Motor Performance and Its Measurement

We will first discuss motor performance, motor skills, and how they are measured in children and adults. Next we will discuss relation between such measures and normal personality variation. We will continue by discussing what little evidence there is for changes of motor performance in mental illnesses.

[1] Preparation of this chapter was supported in part by training grants from the National Institute of Mental Health (MH-16880) and from the National Institute of Child Health and Human Development (HD-07289). I appreciate the expert editorial assistance of Rebecca G. Miles.

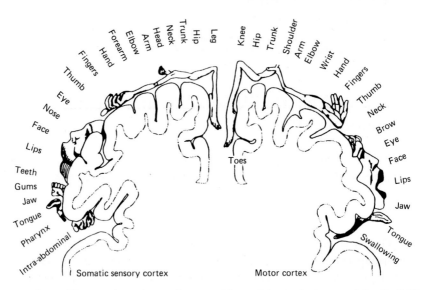

Fig. 1. The somatic sensory and motor regions of the cerebral cortex (after Penfield). [Reprinted from Smyth and Wing, 1984, p. 34, with permission.]

We will start with a brief summary of the physiology and neural control of movement. Most of the readers will remember the homunculus representation of the motor regions of the cerebral cortex shown in figure 1 and they may also remember that the cerebellum controls many functions which are largely automatic, i.e., outside of our conscious control. Damage to the part called the neocerebellum impairs voluntary movements. Feedback from the sensory areas is extremely important in all movement. For our purposes it is not necessary to go further into the nervous control of movement. For an introduction into this area a book edited by Smyth and Wing [1984] entitled *The Psychology of Human Movement* can be recommended. For more detailed treatment, reference can be made to the chapters in the book edited by Kandel and Schwartz [1981], especially the chapter entitled 'Introduction to the motor systems'. Also useful are chapters in the 1960 *Handbook of Physiology* especially section I, *Neurophysiology* volume 2, edited by Magoun, and the twentieth edition of *Physiology and Biophysics: The Brain and Neural Function* [Ruch and Patton, 1974]. From the older work two citations from the chapter 'The general principles of motor integration' by Denny-Brown [1960, p. 393] are worth quoting:

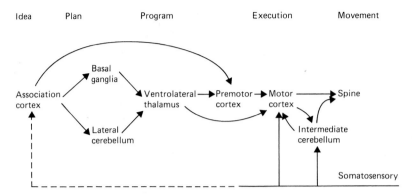

Fig. 2. Hypothetical relations between brain structure and voluntary movement. [Reprinted from Smyth and Wing, 1984, p. 296, with permission.]

'Two important general principles emerge. First, every motor reaction has an adequate stimulus, immediate or remote; and second, all that is known of motor function indicates that *the nervous system as a whole contributes to each motor act*. It is not possible to indicate separate mechanisms for posture and movement. Postural reactions are fundamental in neural organization, and movement in its most elementary form is seen as modifications of postural responses. There is a similar difficulty in defining "function" which can be used only in a general sense equivalent to activity. The operative physiological term is "performance" which from spinal to cortical levels can be traced in various grades of refinement and in more appropriate relation to the whole organism and finally the whole environment.

It is the *cerebral cortex* with its projections of the exteroceptors, that *dominates the whole*, able to select items of behavior and modify them in terms of projected reactions. There are only very slender clues as to the mechanism of cortical domination.'

These statements emphasize the close, intricate connection between motor behavior and cognition including personality.

One finds little or no mention of individual differences in texts about the nervous system with the important exception of abnormal motor behavior which is the domain of neurology. A brief introduction to disorders of movement is offered by Wing [1984]. The interesting diagram (fig. 2) from that chapter shows the many steps from the formation of an idea to the execution of a movement. At each of these steps damage will result in impairment. This will not be discussed here nor is there any attempt to cover development in infants of motor behavior to which Gesell and Amatruda [1941] made such basic contributions. Finally, it is beyond my capacity to relate this to the work of child neurologists such as Prechtl [Connolly and

Prechtl, 1981; Touwen and Prechtl, 1970]. Instead we turn to the later individual differences in the normal range of movements which have been studied under the rubrics of motor skills, physical fitness, and learning. Much of this work has been hampered by the lack of agreement on the tests to be used or the skills to be measured. The Bayley infant tests [Bayley, 1969] include a number of motor items, but this motor information is not usually followed up. Oseretsky [1929, 1931] proposed a battery for use with older children measuring, according to him, the following six components with his idea about their various control:

(a) *General static coordination:* This component is conceptualized as a general ability to keep one's balance while standing still, which presumes the intactness of the cerebellar systems and the vestibular and other sensory apparatus connected with the cerebellum.

(b) *Dynamic manual coordination* and

(c) *General dynamic coordination:* These two components were apparently separated from Gurewitsch's original concept of dynamic coordination [Gurewitsch and Oseretsky, 1925], which was concerned with balance while in motion, the maintenance of direction of motion, as well as the smooth timing of innervation and denervation. Gurewitsch considered this component to be under the control of all motoric systems of the brain, but particularly of the frontal cerebellar mechanisms.

(d) *Speed of movements:* This component is thought to be due to a complex combination of tempo (under the control of striate mechanisms and activated by the frontal-thalamic system), the innervation-denervation cycle (striocerebellar system) and the degree of development of automatized motor responses (localized in the cortex). All of these, in addition, are under some control of the higher motoric centers.

(e) *Ability to perform simultaneous movement* (with more than one extremity) dependent on the highest motoric cortical centers.

(f) *Absence of synkinesia* (or superfluous side movements) is also considered under the control of cortical motor centers.

Factor analyses of the item correlations by Thams [1955] and by Vandenberg [1964] failed to show correspondence between the empirical factors and the components proposed by Oseretsky. Other batteries for children have been published by Van Der Lugt [1949] and Yarmolenko [1933]. There are numerous tests of more limited scope such as tests of physical fitness or of specific sports skills. See for instance Barrow and McGee [1964] for a list of 45 tests for golf, badminton, basketball, etc. Another long list can be found in Mathews [1973].

Most measures of adult intelligence have not included motor performances items. Fleishman has performed research on motor skill differences in
adults for many years and has suggested a number of factors underlying
motor skills. In 1954, Fleishman suggested the following 10 independent
interpretable factors: (1) finger-wrist speed; (2) finger dexterity; (3) rate of
arm movement; (4) aiming; (5) arm-hand steadiness; (6) reaction time;
(7) manual dexterity; (8) psychomotor speed; (9) psychomotor coordination, and (10) spatial relationship.

In 1984, Fleishman and Quaintance summarized 11 psychomotor factors as well as 9 physical proficiency factors, all shown in table I. Of course,
these factors depend on the tasks selected for inclusion. Although only a
weak general factor has been found in normal individuals, one might expect
to find a larger general difference between normal and mental patients, just
as is the case with mental retardation. We shall see later if there is any
evidence for such a tendency.

Since no one general factor suffices to describe motor performance, it
becomes less likely that one will find a single strong relationship of motoric
behavior with personality traits, except possibly where personality traits such
as motivation or anxiety act as moderator variables.

Since 1965 there exists an international committee for the standardization of physical fitness tests. They have worked in a different tradition for the
measurement of fitness and work capacity, a tradition closer to the physiology and biochemistry of the muscle. This tradition ignores or is critical of the
factor analytic work, probably because they question its usefulness and
especially the lack of a theoretical foundation based on physiology. A good
exposition of this alternate approach may be found in a book by the international committee, edited by Larson [1974], or a more recent book by Berger
[1982]. For summary, see table II and figure 3.

The distinction between Fleishman's work and this second approach is
somewhat reminiscent of the split between classical experimental psychology,
which tends to emphasize single variables that are studied under as closely
controlled conditions as possible, and the multivariate, individual differences
approach in psychology.

An additional plus of the single-measurement-at-one-time approach has
been that it has been able to consider the size and shape of the body in order
to predict the performance of an individual better. In fact it was possible to
calculate the exact amount of energy expended in calories by top athletes in
their peak performances (fig. 4).

The energy derives from several sources. It is not possible to go into any

Table I. Psychomotor and physical proficiency factors resulting from Fleishman's factor analytic studies [reprinted from Fleishman and Quaintance, 1984, pp. 164–166, with permission]

Psychomotor Factors

Control Precision
The ability to make fine, highly controlled muscular movements required to adjust the position of a control mechanism. Examples of control mechanisms are joysticks, levels, pedals, and rudders. A series of adjustments may be required, but they need not be performed simultaneously. This ability is most critical where adjustments must be rapid, but precise. Adjustments are made to visual stimuli and involve the use of a single limb, either arm-hand or leg.
Examples: *Rotary Pursuit Test; operate a joystick to steer an aircraft.*

Multilimb Coordination
The ability to coordinate the movement of a number of limbs simultaneously. Best measured by devices involving multiple controls (hands, feet, or hands and feet).
Examples: *Complex Coordination Test; operate a bulldozer.*

Response Orientation
This factor is general to visual discrimination tasks. These tasks involve rapid recognition of the direction (north, south, east, west) indicated by a particular visual stimulus (e.g., an arrow) followed by the appropriate motor response chosen from several alternatives. The response may be simple or complex (push a button and pull a switch vs. push a button). This ability appears to be most critical when the conditions are highly speeded.
Example: *Flip different switches in response to different colored lights appearing on a display panel.*

Reaction Time
This ability represents the speed with which the individual can provide a single motor response to a single stimulus when it appears. It is independent of the mode of presentation (auditory or visual) and also of the type of motor response required. Response cannot involve alternate choices.
Example: *Depress a button as soon as possible after hearing a buzzer.*

Speed of Arm Movement
The speed with an individual can make a gross, discrete arm movement where accuracy is minimized. There is ample evidence that this ability is independent of reaction time.
Example: *Move a series of control levers to new positions in rapid succession.*

Rate Control
Involves the timing of continuous anticipatory motor adjustments relative to changes in speed and/or direction of a continuously moving target or object. Actual motor response to change (rather than a verbal stimulus) is necessary. Extends to tasks involving compensatory as well as following pursuit and to those involving responses to changes in rate.
Example: *Track a moving target by keeping a circle around a dot which changes in speed and direction of movement.*

Manual Dexterity
The ability to make skillful, well-directed arm-hand movements in manipulating fairly large objects under speeded conditions.
Examples: *Minnesota Rate of Manipulation Test; use hand tools to assemble an aircraft engine.*

Table I (continued)

Psychomotor Factors

Finger Dexterity
The ability to make skillful, controlled manipulations of objects small enough to be handled with the fingers.
Examples: *Purdue Pegboard Test; assemble peg, washer, and collar units and insert them in small holes.*

Arm-Hand Steadiness
The ability to make precise arm-hand positioning movements in which strength and speed are minimized. It extends to tasks that require steadiness during movement as well as those that require a minimum of tremor while maintaining a static arm position.
Examples: *Arm Tremor Test; perform retinal surgery.*

Wrist-Finger Speed
The ability to make rapid pendular (back and forth) and/or rotary wrist movements in which accuracy is not critical.
Example: *Tapping Test.*

Aiming
The ability to make highly accurate, restricted hand movements requiring precise eye-hand coordination.
Example: *Make a dot in a series of very small circles on a printed test.*

Physical Proficiency Factors

Extent Flexibility
The ability to extend or stretch the body. Tests that load on this factor require stretching of the trunk and back muscles as far as possible, without speed, either laterally, forward, or backward.
Example: *Twist as far around as possible, touching the scale on the wall.*

Dynamic Flexibility
Common to tasks that require rapid and repeated trunk and/or limb movements. Emphasizes both speed and flexibility.
Example: *Without moving your feet, bend and touch a spot on the floor, stand up, twist, and touch a spot on the wall behind as rapidly as possible.*

Explosive Strength
Common to tasks that require expenditure of a maximum of energy in one or a series of explosive acts. This factor emphasizes the mobilization of energy for a burst of effort, rather than continuous strain, stress, or repeated extertion of muscles.
Examples: *Broad jump; sprint 50 yards.*

Static Strength
Common to tasks that require the exertion of maximum strength against a fairly immovable external object, even for a brief period. It is general to different muscle groups (hand, arm, back, shoulder, leg) and to different kinds ot tasks.
Examples: *Squeeze a grip dynamometer as hard as possible; lift heavy objects.*

Table I (continued)

Physical Proficiency Factors

Dynamic Strength
The ability to exert muscular force repeatedly or continuously over time. It represents muscular endurance and emphasizes the resistance of the muscles to fatigue. Tests loading on this factor tend to emphasize the power of the muscles to propel, support, or move the body repeatedly or the support it for prolonged periods.
Examples: *Pull-ups; scale a wall.*

Trunk Strength
This is a second, more limited, dynamic strength factor specific to the trunk muscles, particularly the abdominal muscles.
Examples: *Leg-lifts; sit-ups.*

Gross Body Coordination
The ability to perform movements simultaneously that involve the entire body.
Example: *Holding the ends of a short rope in each hand, jump over the rope without tripping, falling or releasing the rope.*

Gross Body Equilibrium
The ability to maintain or regain body balance, especially in situations in which equilibrium is theatened or temporarily lost.
Example: *Walk a narrow rail without falling off.*

Stamina (Cardiovascular Endurance)
The ability to exert sustained physical effort involving the cardiovascular system.
Examples: *Run a distance of one mile as fast as you can; extinguish a building fire.*

Comments: It will be necessary to develop a selection of these tasks for a mentally ill patient so that their cooperation can be maximized.

---

details here. Suffice it to say that the most important distinction is between what are called aerobic and anaerobic processes. The first derives its energy from the oxidation of glycogen (or glucose) to allow the splitting of adenosine triphosphate (ATP), adenosine diphosphate (ADP) or phosphocreatinine (PC) to produce high energy phosphate (P), which in turn produces the 'fuel' for the electrical discharges that produce the brief contractions of the muscle spindles. This output can vary from the single concentrated explosion of the spectacular leap of a male ballet dancer to the sustained effort of the long distance runner or bicycle rider. In most cases where more than the ordinary routine effort is involved a second class of chemical processes take over. Speaking in an exaggerated way we might almost say that in these

Table II. Physical performance components: their definitions and measurements [reprinted from Berger, 1982, p.244, with permission]

Component	Operational definition	Measurement
Absolute strength	strength in moving a heavy object other than body weight or applying force to an immovable object	maximum force applied to an external object, such as a barbell, in movement (concentric contraction) or a dynamometer (isometric contraction)
Relative strength	strength in moving body weight or strength per pound of body weight	chins, dips, push-ups, rope climb, or any measure where maximum number of repetitions with body weight is less than about 25
Absolute power	strength or force in moving an external weight quickly and explosively	medicine ball put, lifting an external load rapidly, and leg power test are examples
Relative power	strength or force in moving body weight quickly and explosively (sometimes referred to as speed when running in one direction, or agility and coordination when running around obstacles)	standing broad jump, vertical jump, shuttle run, dodge run, 50-yard dash, softball throw, and 10-yard dash are examples
Aerobic endurance	endurance in moving large muscle groups repeatedly for 3 min or more, but preferably for over 5 min; the limitations in performance are primarily in the oxygen delivery system and at the cellular level	all-out running, swimming, or cycling for more than 3 min;
Anaerobic-aerobic endurance	endurance in moving large muscle groups repeatedly for at least 1 min, but not for more than 2 min; the limitations in performance lie within the muscles' shortterm energy supply and the oxygen delivery system	all-out running, swimming, or cycling for 1–3 min
Relative muscular endurance	endurance is repeatedly lifting body weight or a light load that is a proportion of maximum strength, by concentric contractions, or sustaining these loads by an isometric contraction; the limitations in performance reside primarily within the muscle itself	performance tests that permit more than 25 repetitions using body weight or an external load that is the same relative load for everyone; sit-ups and leg raises are examples of appropriate tests; also, maintaining a sustained isometric contraction for more than about 60 s, such as in a bent arm chin, is an effective measurement
Absolute muscular endurance	endurance in repeatedly lifting an external weight or in sustaining it by an isometric contraction	performance tests that permit more than 25 repetitions with loads that are the same for all testees

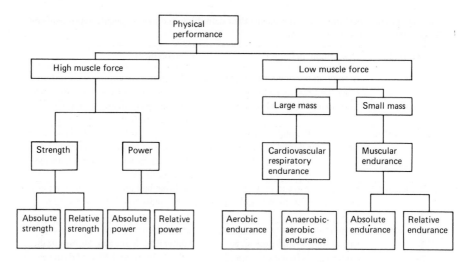

Fig. 3. A model of physical performance. [Reprinted from Berger, 1982, p. 242, with permission.]

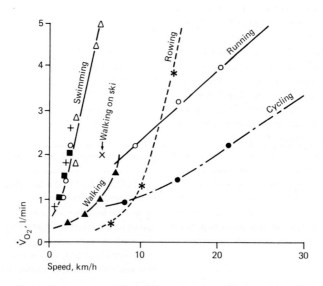

Fig. 4. Oxygen uptake (liter/min) as a function of the speed (km/h) for different exercises: + = underwater swimming: o = back stroke: ■ = breast stroke: △ = crawl; * = data refer to energy expenditure of a single rower in a 'two with coxswain' shell. [Reprinted from Cerretelli, 1974, p. 132, with permission.]

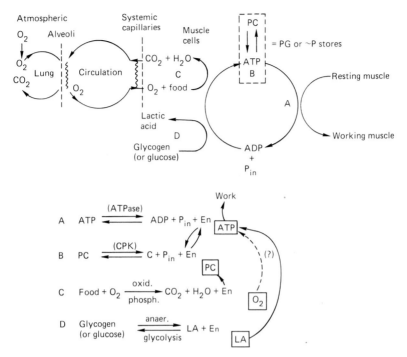

Fig. 5. Schematic representation of the various energy sources for muscular work. A, B, C und D correspond to the different reactions as indicated in the modified Lohmann scheme above. [Reprinted from Cerretelli, 1974, p. 113, with permission.]

efforts the muscles themselves are destroyed by the anaerobic conversion of glycogen to lactic acid. This process is usually subjectively experienced by the athlete as very painful, so that runners and swimmers for example speak of fighting through it. Substantial amounts of the total energy used in athletic feats of strength and endurance come from these latter processes and account for the longer recovery periods compared to the relatively short period of breathlessness due to the increased consumption of oxygen during the feat. However, the term 'oxygen debt' is not used solely to refer to that breathless period, but is also used to describe the continued increased need for oxygen (compared to the normal resting condition) due to the necessity for 'repair', i.e. to reconvert lactic acid back to glycogen. See figure 5 for a schematic representation of these processes.

Such precise calculations are possible that generalizations have been made about the optimal combinations of body type and physical perform-

Table III. Relation between body size and athletic performance [from Morehouse and Rasch, 1964 with permission]

Body height	Body weight	Sport	
		men	women
Tall	heavy	heavyweight boxing football end football tackle heavyweight wrestling	field hockey goalie soccer goalie lacrosse
Tall	medium	discus thrower, javelin thrower basketball center basketball pitcher	modern dance softball pitcher volleyball
Tall	light	high jumper, hurdler tennis middle-distance runner fencing cross-country runner	tennis basketball softball, first base
Medium	heavy	shot putter football fullback football guard, tackle, or center	speedball archery bowling
Medium	medium	distance swimming golf bowling	swimming field hockey forward golf synchronized swimmers
Medium	light	distance runner badminton baseball second baseman lightweight boxer	fencing badminton softball infielder
Short	heavy	baseball catcher ice hockey defense weight lifter	softball catcher backfield-soccer backfield-hockey
Short	medium	gymnastic apparatus handball springboard diver water polo guard	diving skiing figure skater
Short	light	soccer forward tumbling figure skater jockey	tap-dancing tumbling soccer forward

Table IV. Factors limiting motor performance

Lung factors
1 Alveolar ventilations
2 Diffusion of the respiratory gases through the alveolocapillary membrane (transfer factor)
Blood factors
3 Oxygen and carbon dioxide uptake by the blood
Cardiocirculatory factors
4 Thoracic circulation (cardiac output)
5 Peripheral circulation
Tissue factors
6 Diffusion of oxygen from the capillaries to the cells
7 Oxygen utilization ability of the cell

ance features in various sports. Table III shows some of these; see also the extended discussion in Berger [1982].

Finally, in the last resort it is the fatty tissues that provide the long range reserves of energy, which may take weeks of starvation to deplete. However, because oxygen plays such a crucial role, all the factors that can affect the ready supply of oxygen (or air) play a role in the capacity for work and effort in sports. Table IV summarizes some of these. Various forms of anemia are interesting as they may not be noted until a major effort at strength or endurance is attempted.

Relation of Motor Performance to Personality

As mentioned before, the physiology of movement is complicated: Control of movement is exerted at many levels and is closely monitored by visual and proprioceptive feedback, so that any injury at one of many levels and places may affect the smoothness and precision of movement. This is why, besides the major disorders of movement, so many other physical diseases affect motor performance [Lockwood et al., 1988; Wing, 1984]. Yet in the majority of cases, the motor proficiency of institutionalized and noninstitutionalized mentally retarded children does not differ much from that of normal children [Malpass, 1960], nor do intellectually gifted children differ from normal children in that respect [McKernon, 1956]. Because mental illness does not appear till later in life, we do not know much about the early motor development of individuals with various types of mental illness, but

Fish [1975] maintained that schizophrenics were frequently awkward and clumsy in childhood. If depression and schizophrenia can be regarded as extremes of normal personality dimensions, then evidence for a relation of personality with motor skills and athletic skills would be valuable in this regard. More about that later.

For the purposes of this chapter, personality will be defined as a complex set of traits and we will accept scores on a wide variety of personality inventories as indicators of such traits. While there is some convergence among the traits measured by the various questionnaires, it is not possible to adhere to one system in what follows. Of course, it would be invaluable for future research if more consensus could be achieved.

One general remark seems in order. One can regard mental illnesses as extremes of the normal distribution of personality traits or as entirely different entities. Both points of view have been taken by various individuals. Eysenck, for instance, developed his questionnaires by contrasting neurotics and psychotics, yet the resulting scales have been used to characterize normal individuals. For the Extraversion-Introversion and the Neuroticism Scales this seems to work rather well, but it has led to problems of interpretation with the Psychoticism Scale. Similarly, the MMPI was developed from the responses chosen by patients, but is also used with normals. In contrast, the scales of Cattell, Comrey, Edwards, Gough, Guilford, Jackson, Leary, Lorr, Tellegen, and others were developed from the responses of normal individuals and then applied, at times, to patients.

What little we know about motor behavior and personality comes from two sources: (a) sport psychology such as studies of the personality of various athletes and (b) speculation based on the limited information from studies of the personalities of people in various jobs and with various leisure time activities.

The field of sport psychology, while not new, has only recently been acknowledged by American psychology in a chapter in the *Annual Review of Psychology* [Browne and Mahoney, 1984]. Perusal of that chapter indicates that the surface has only been scratched, and except for some interesting hints, little of a systematic theory exists. The most meaningful relationship found so far is that between Zuckerman's Sensation-Seeking Scales [Zuckerman, 1979], extraversion, and certain types of sports. A problem with much of the research in the area of sport psychology is that general conclusions are drawn from small samples of athletes which are formed, of necessity, by rather selected individuals who are not necessarily representative of the general population or even of all participants in that sport [Kirkcaldy, 1985].

Table V. Means, standard deviations, and univariate F values for hang gliders, automobile racers, and bowlers on Zuckerman's Sensation-Seeking Scale (Form V) [adapted from Straub, 1982, p. 249, with permission]

Test compo-nent	Hang gliders (n = 33)		Auto racers (n = 22)		Bowlers (n = 25)		F value
	mean	SD	mean	SD	mean	SD	
Thrill and adventure seeking	8.12	1.92	7.41	2.56	6.28	2.68	4.35*
Experience seeking	5.42	2.26	5.18	1.84	3.56	2.27	5.83**
Disinhibitions	5.06	3.04	5.73	2.19	4.40	2.16	1.56
Boredom susceptibility	2.67	1.95	4.32	1.89	3.16	1.77	5.17**
First compo-nent	21.27	2.29	22.64	2.12	17.40	2.22	3.79*

* $p < 0.05$; ** $p < 0.01$.

Yet it is important to know how athletes of various types really differ from nonathletes and from one another in one or more aspects.

Many findings tend to confirm popular stereotypes. Confirmed counter-intuitive findings would be much more impressive. We cannot attempt to review all studies but only some suggestive ones.

Pestonje et al. [1981] compared 46 individuals (29 boys and 17 girls) who were involved in sports and physical activities with another group of 29 boys and 17 girls who were not involved in such activities. The results with the Cattell 16 PF test suggested that the sports group were more socially oriented, more confident, and less interested in ideas than the other group. This was especially true for the boys.

Kirkcaldy [1982] reported that offensive (attacking) players in male team sports were more tough-minded, dominant, and aggressive (Eysenck's P factor) and more extraverted than midfield players. Those in defensive positions were less emotional (neurotic) than the offensive players but did not differ on the other two dimensions. For women, attacking players were less extraverted and more emotional (neurotic) than midfield or backfield players.

Straub [1982] tested 33 male hang gliders, 22 automobile racers, and 25 intercollegiate bowlers with Zuckerman's Sensation-Seeking Scale. His results, shown in table V, suggest that the first two groups do differ from the third. The auto racers had the highest total score followed by the hang gliders.

Maier and Lavrakas [1981] reported that in a sample of 71 male undergraduates of Loyola University, certain traditional, masculine role attitudes were related to attitudes about winning at all costs, about the place of women in sports and about physical contact sports.

Burke [1986] compared androgyny scores on the Benn androgyny inventory of 11 basketball players, 12 softball players, 17 swimmers, and 9 tennis players (all female) and found a small (p <0.05) increase in masculinity for the first two compared to the last two groups.

A very interesting book introduced another aspect of sports. Csikszentmihaly [1975] described how absorption in some activities can lead to a special mental condition, named by him as the 'flow experience', in which one loses the sense of the passage of time and of one's self. In some ways this experience resembles ecstacy as described in the book by Laski [1961]. This experience can occur in chess as well as in rock climbing so it is total concentration rather than the physical activity that is responsible. The work by Csikszentmihaly suggests that there may be relationships between recreational interests and personality, just as there are relationships between vocational interests and personality as for instance, worked out by Holland [1966], for the individual differences found between occupations in the scores of the Strong Vocational Interest Scales. It will be remembered that Holland has proposed that the underlying structure can be thought of as hexagonal. The six orientations are summarized by Holland [1966] as follows:

(1) *Realistic:* The model type is masculine, physically strong, unsociable, aggressive; has good motor coordination and skill; lacks verbal and interpersonal skills; prefers concrete to abstract problems; conceives of himself as being aggressive and masculine and as having conventional political and economic values. Persons who choose or prefer the following occupations resemble this type: airplane mechanic, electrician, filling station attendant, fish and wildlife specialist, master plumber, photoengraver, surveyor, and tool designer, etc.

(2) *Intellectual:* The model type is task-oriented, intraceptive, asocial; prefers to think through rather than act out problems; needs to understand; enjoys ambiguous work tasks; has unconventional values and attitudes; is anal as opposed to oral. Vocational preferences include aeronautical design engineer, anthropologist, biologist, chemist, geologist, physicist, and scientific research worker, etc.

(3) *Social:* The model type is sociable, responsible, feminine, humanistic, religious; needs attention; has verbal and interpersonal skills; avoids intellectual problem-solving, physical activity, and highly ordered activities; prefers to solve problems through feelings and interpersonal manipulations of others; is orally dependent. Vocational preferences include assistant city school superintendent, clinical psychologist, director of welfare agency, high school teacher, physical education teacher, psychiatric case worker, social science teacher, and vocational counselor.

(4) *Conventional:* The model type prefers structured verbal and numerical activities and subordinate roles; is conforming (extraceptive); avoids ambiguous situations and problems involving interpersonal relationships and physical skills; is effective at well-structured tasks; identifies with power; values material possessions and status. Vocational preferences include: bank examiner, bookkeeper, court stenographer, financial analyst, payroll clerk, statistician, and traffic manager.

(5) *Enterprising:* The model type has verbal skills for selling, dominating, leading; conceives of himself as a strong, masculine leader; avoids well-defined language or work situations requiring long periods of intellectual effort; is extraceptive; differs from the Conventional type in that he prefers ambiguous social tasks and has a greater concern with power, status, and leadership; is orally aggressive. Vocational preferences include business executive, industrial relations' consultant, political campaign manager, real-estate salesman, restaurant worker, sports promotor, and television producer, etc.

(6) *Artistic:* The model type is asocial; avoids problems that are highly structured or require gross physical skills, resembles the intellectual type in being intraceptive and asocial, but differs from that type in that he has a need for individualistic expression, has less ego strength, is more feminine, and suffers more frequently from emotional disturbances; prefers dealing with environmental problems through self-expression in artistic media. Vocational preferences include art dealer, author, commercial artist, concert singer, freelance writer, musician, poet, and symphony conductor.

Unfortunately the Strong Vocational Interest Blank does not include a scoring key (or keys) for professional athletes, whether they play tennis, golf, football, basketball, or even bowling. For that reason, it is not possible to guess where they would fall in Holland's scheme. Indications from recreational interests on sports activities of nonprofessional players may help.

Although Holland derived his six types mainly from research based on the Strong Vocational Interest Blank which was developed for applied (vocational guidance) purposes, some of the six types bear a remarkable similarity to the six basic life orientations described by Spranger [1921] on an intuitive basis. These six life-styles are: *Theoretical, Economic, Aesthetic, Social, Political,* and *Religious,* and formed the basis for the Allport-Vernon-Lindzey scale of values. It may have occurred to the reader that the Holland vocational typology also bears some resemblance to the complex model of interpersonal behavior of Leary [1957], Foa [1961], Schulz [1958], Lorr and McNair [1965a, b], and Wiggins [1973]. We will see later that the same holds for McKechnie's recreational types, and the Bolles' model of recreation.

Wiggins' interpersonal behavior model, shown in figure 6, is based on ideas of Sullivan [1953], who proposed two orthogonal axes: *power* (dominance versus submission) and *affiliation* (love versus hate). Note the similarity of those axes to Earl Schaefer's dimensions of parental behavior [Schaefer, 1966]. It is not clear how this model can be related to Eysenck's three or four higher order personality factors of Neuroticism, Extraversion-Introversion, Psychoticism, and the Lie Scale.

We mentioned that recreational activities may be related to personality differences in ways similar to occupational types. It so happens that in the data based on a sample of 286 subjects used by McKechnie for the development of the Leisure Activities Blank there are frequent hints at relationships between personality traits and sports activities. For that reason we will describe this instrument in some detail.

Because of the clear practical applications of vocational scales for counseling, Strong devoted most of his career to the improvement and promotion of his interest scale. In contrast, the study of recreational interests has lagged behind. Perhaps the best work has been done by McKechnie [1972, 1974]. He constructed a 120-item Leisure Activities Blank which is scored for the following 6 scales: (1) *Mechanics;* (2) *Crafts;* (3) *Intellectual;* (4) *Slow Living;* (5) *Sports,* and (6) *Glamour Sports.* This first part of the inventory relates to past experiences. The second part deals with recreation projected into future plans and uses the same 120 items, but is scored for 8 scales: (1) *Adventure;* (2) *Mechanics;* (3) *Crafts;* (4) *Easy Living;* (5) *Intellectual;* (6) *Ego Recognition;* (7) *Slow Living,* and (8) *Clean Living.* The similarity of some of the latter scales to the 6 past scales indicates some continuity in the grouping of interests, but it is clear that future research will have to give more attention to age differences and the development of and changes in a person's interests or in the role of reinforcements and opportunities. Furthermore, it seems unlikely that the interests of males and females will be found to be sufficiently similar to permit the use of exactly the same instrument.

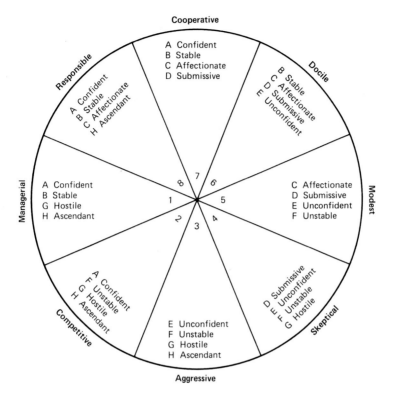

Fig. 6. The interpersonal circumplex, based on the ideas of Sullivan [1953] and Wiggins [1973], among others. [Reprinted from Wiggins, 1973, p. 480, with permission.]

This resembles the situation with respect of the Strong scales where a common set of scales for men and women were eventually developed. While the manual for the McKechnie LAB gives some correlations with other tests such as the Strong, the California Psychological Inventory and the Study of Values, no effort has been made to look for an underlying structure of interest factors and to relate such a structure to broader personality traits. It seems likely that differences in intelligence and in socioeconomic levels would complicate such a relationship.

The research required to explore these complications will probably not be undertaken until the demands of recreation and sports counselors will make it more than an interesting theoretical area of research. The McKechnie scales are summarized as follows:

Mechanics–Past

ME (past) summary: High past involvement in mechanics activities identifies a person who is masculine, sociable but not warm or compassionate, and very practical minded. He appears to enjoy interacting with people on a friendly, informal basis, but shies away from the deeper psychological aspects of life: close emotional involvement or self-reflection. At his worst, he may be hypermasculine: crude, egotistical, hardheaded, power-oriented. The person scoring low on the mechanics' cluster, in contrast, is more open to the emotional aspects of life, aesthetically responsive, and responsible. At his worst, however, he exhibits a touchiness and preoccupation with his own problems.

Crafts–Past

CR (past) summary: Aside from the obvious sex-role component of Crafts, high scorers are emotional persons. This emotionality may appear as a fickle, spunky, impulsive pattern that is at once independent and immature. But the high scorer is also compassionate, aesthetically responsive, and natural. Strong involvement in crafts appears to represent a displacement of much psychic energy – energy otherwise destined to support strong and enduring emotional relationships – into the creation of domestic artifacts which symbolize warmth, concern, and devotion. Low scores on Crafts are indicative of a person who is calm, deliberate, logical, and mannerly: in a word, stolid. The strength of this psychological configuration is stability and planfulness; what it lacks is spontaneity and verve.

Intellectual–Past

IN (past) summary: The intellectual cluster taps interest and ability in ideational matters. High scorers are dominant, have wide interests, are active, sophisticated, and somewhat selfish. In leisure activities, these people put their brains before their bodies. They are accustomed to assertive action in their personal lives, and this style carries over into their recreation patterns. This self-contained and self-possessed quality may make them unrealistic in their expectations of other people. Low scorers tend to be conventional, conservative, easygoing, and perhaps a bit dull. Their strengths, however, include friendliness, patience, and joviality.

Slow Living–Past

SL (past) summary: The slow living cluster is the province of planful individuals. They are healthy and good-looking persons who value their own

independence. Leisure for these persons is the payoff for efficient and energetic work effort, a time to slow down, relax, and do nothing constructive
other than simple enjoyment of life. At the other end of the Slow Living
Scale is a configuration that might best be described as: neurotic, awkward,
contented, self-denying, self-pitying. Low scorers have a poor self-image,
perhaps related to what they perceive to be below-average physical appearance. They feel undeserving, and thus deny themselves the simple everyday
indulgences of the Slow Living Scale.

Sports–Past

SP (past) summary: Sports activities are competitive, and high scorers
are well aware of this fact. They are dominant, foresighted, achievement-
oriented, ambitious, even opportunistic and aggressive individuals. They
know what they want and have the wherewithall to attain it. The motivation
here is to compete and win, even at the expense of other persons. Power is all
important. At the same time, however, they are sociable, tolerant, and well-
adjusted. They judge it acceptable and even good for others to have similar
goals and aspirations. This is all part of the game. Low scores on SP reflect
concern with aesthetic and philosophical matters. These qualities may be
seen by others as reflecting weakness and immobility.

Glamour Sports–Past

GS (past) summary: High scorers on Glamour Sports display social
ascendency, spontaneity, the ability to enjoy themselves, tolerance, flexibility
and optimism. They are aware of their own social impact on other persons,
and are likely to be attentive to a variety of social status cues. Low scorers on
GS, in contrast, are a gloomy lot. They appear to be preoccupied with their
own personal problems and situation in life, and are unable to respond
effectively or adaptively to the opportunities for enjoyable leisure that the
glamor sports activities provide.

Adventure–Future

AD (future) summary: High scores are indicative of high social presence, effective intellectual functioning, alert and energetic adventure, and
irresponsible, perhaps occasionally reckless, action. Persons who express
interest in adventure activities are imaginative, opportunistic, and sensuous.
Low scorers are stolid, stern, rigid, retiring, conservative, withdrawing, and
moralistic.

Mechanics–Future

ME (future) summary: Anticipation of future mechanics activity, like actual past participation in Mechanics behaviors, connotes an orientation toward the physical rather than the psychological world. High scorers on ME (Future) are concerned with practical matters and facts. Although they enjoy doing things with other people, this sociability does *not* extend to the point where they are willing to become emotionally involved with or take responsibility for the acts of others. They are interested in getting ahead in life, and this quality may be seen by others as coarse, opportunistic, or self-seeking behavior. The low scorer on ME (Future), in contrast, is interested in aesthetics and matters of the mind, and is seen by others as undercontrolled, retiring, and perhaps even weak.

Crafts–Future

CR (future) summary: Much like the CR (past) cluster, CR (future) taps a personality configuration defined by aesthetic interests, femininity, personal warmth, and openness to unconventional thoughts and ideas. Also present, however, are components of self-sacrifice, distractibility, and idealism. Low scores, on the other hand, connote a conservative, assertive, power-oriented configuration. Low scorers are described as stolid, unemotional, deliberate, and mannerly.

Easy Living–Future

EL (future) summary: People who work in a world of objects and actions (e.g., veterinarian, production manager, credit manager) rather than with abstract ideas (e.g., psychologist, biologist, mathematician) tend to express interest in EL (future) activities. The high scorer on EL is sociable, outgoing, practical, and optimistic. He is concerned with achievement and adopts economic and political value orientations. The low scorer, in contrast, is introspective, introverted, aloof, perhaps even withdrawn. He is concerned with philosophical problems in life, and has adopted an aesthetic value orientation.

Intellectual–Future

IN (future) summary: Individuals who express an interest in these activities desire to mix work with pleasure. High scorers have administrative interests and are verbally fluent and insightful. They are alert, tactful, and enjoy social interaction. For these people, their work *is* their pleasure. Low scorers, in contrast, are retiring, simple, silent, perhaps even awkward. They are less oriented to matters of intellectual expression and interpersonal involvement than to direct action in an inanimate world.

Ego Recognition–Future

ER (future) summary: This cluster of activities taps a youthful and typically masculine pattern of personality functioning: adventurous, outgoing, daring, and uninhibited. The high scorer is a show-off. He may use his considerable social skills to deceive or manipulate, to stretch limits, and perhaps to act out sexual impulses. The low scorer, in contrast, is described as lazy, relaxed, and conservative.

Slow Living–Future

SL (future) summary: Anticipation of future SL activities is related to hustle and physical and psychological well-being in one's present life. The high scorer on this cluster is high on personal adjustment, makes a good impression on others, and is concerned with his adequacy as a person. He works hard at life, and looks forward to a time when he can sit back, relax, and reap the rewards of his efforts. In contrast, low scorers are described as contented, absentminded, forgetful, and retiring. They may also be subject to depressive or repressive reactions.

Clean Living–Future

CL (future) summary: This cluster of leisure activities connotes an extroverted, sociable personality type. High scorers on CL are described as enthusiastic, friendly, optimistic, and wholesome. Low scorers, on the other hand, are absentminded, reflective, confused, and introverted. They have aesthetic interests, and, like the SL (future) low scorers, are prone to depressive and repressive responses.

Before the detailed description of the McKechnie scales, mention was made of the absence of a higher order structure. In an interesting book by Bolles [1973] a speculative scheme for ordering leisure time activities is provided (fig. 7). It may be seen that the vertical axis runs from 'solitude' to 'being related to other people' and the horizontal runs from 'Spectator' to 'Participant'. It is not clear whether the distance from the center reflects anything else than the position of the activity relative to these two dimensions. It is interesting to note that sexual activity is near the very bottom of the diagram. It is interesting because Eysenck and associates have studied

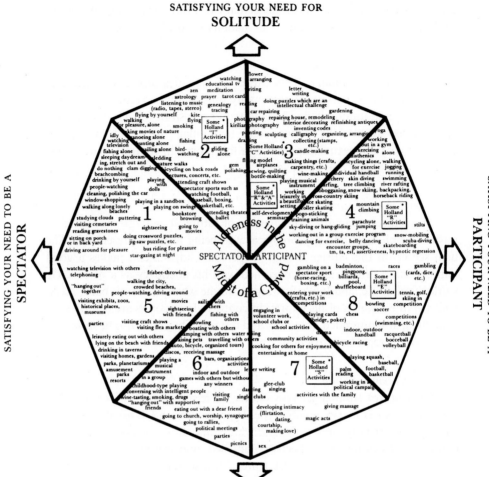
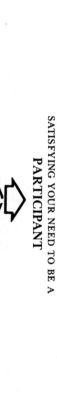

Fig. 7. Map of leisure time activities, similar to Holland's typology of occupations. The three boxes of life, and how to get out of them. [Reprinted from Bolles, 1973, p. 389, with permission.]

personality factors and sexual behavior [Eysenck, 1976; Eysenck and Wilson, 1979]. Sexual behavior is shown by them to be a multivariate phenomenon that cannot be reduced to a simple item in a recreational interests scheme. This research is summarized by Wilson [1986] and critically reviewed by Gilbert [1986, p. 204] who concludes that Eysenck's theory '... suggests that extraverts prefer higher levels of stimulation and have less well-developed consciences than do introverts. These sensation-seeking and socialization factors are seen as working together to predict that extraverts will experience more sexual activity sooner and with more variations and partners than introverts. The high emotional reactivity of individuals scoring high on neuroticism (N) is predicted to cause them to worry more about sex, to be more disgusted by certain sexual acts and to have more sexual inhibitions. The individual scoring high on Eysenck's third personality factor, psychoticism (P), is predicted to be characterized as having an impersonal, cold and aggressive orientation to both sex and life in general.'

A most interesting question that has so far received little attention is whether people enjoy recreational activities that are similar to activities they perform during their working hours or whether they try to compensate in their hobbies for unpleasant aspects of their work and try to contrast the two. The answer seems to differ between types of occupations [Kabanoff, 1980]. Some individuals have stated that their occupation is their recreation and that they do not want to do anything else. Others find their jobs so boring or exhausting that they seek an escape in their leisure activities [Kabanoff and O'Brien, 1980].

Motor Performance and Mental Illness

Rather than looking for relations between normal personality traits and motor skills on the assumption that mental illness is just one or another extreme form of normal personality variation, one can also start at the other end and ask whether there is any direct evidence for changed or diminished motor ability in mentally ill persons. There is little accumulated knowledge about this for obvious reasons. One does not generally inquire about physical skills or minor motor difficulties in psychiatric practice, although a neurologist might do so. We will return to this point when we mention the Nebraska-Luria battery. Yet there was an earlier tradition of experimental work with mental patients strongly influenced by Kretchmer [1936]. Thus it is possible to find the following quotation from 1941:

'Trained observers have long been aware of differences in motor function among psychotics, psychoneurotics and normals. The inability to state these differences in quantitative terms has not destroyed the belief that there are significant modifications resulting from the disease process.'

This is from a paper in which Wulfeck [1941] reported differences between the motor performances of 23 schizophrenics, 25 manic-depressives, 25 neurotics, and 50 normal controls.

In 1973, Yates wrote a chapter on psychomotor deficits in mentally ill patients. He summarized scores on psychomotor differences between normals, neurotics, and psychotics and in a second part of the paper attempted 'to select those factors in an orderly way and evaluate the various theories which have been put forward to account for the facts'. But first he pointed out that in normal subjects most psychomotor tasks are positively but mostly weakly correlated. Thus a general psychomotor ability factor with normals is not useful. Yates further reminded us that subjectivity in scoring plays a far greater role in psychomotor tasks than in cognitive ones.

Few studies of abnormal subjects had used a multivariate approach so Yates' review is mainly of single test measures, generally a different one for each study. Nevertheless, Yates came to four broad conclusions. His final conclusions were as follows:

(1) Compared with normal subjects, neurotics show no significant disorganization on *simple* psychomotor tasks (and may actually do better than normals). They do, however, show marked disorganization compared to normals on *complex* psychomotor tasks. This disorganization is not a function of lower intelligence or poorer special abilities.

(2) Within the total neurotic subgroup, there is evidence that introverted neurotics (i.e. dysthymics) show a different kind of motor disorganization compared with extraverted neurotics (i.e. hysterics); this difference is found also in normal individuals between extraverts and introverts.

(3) Compared with normal subjects, psychotics show significant disorganization on both *simple* and *complex* psychomotor tasks.

(4) There is some evidence that psychomotor tests which discriminate best between neurotics and normals are different from those which discriminate best between psychotics and normals, i.e. that psychosis and neurosis also represent different dimensions in motor performance.

Yates' chapter appeared in a book edited by Eysenck and is clearly influenced by his ideas on personality. It should be noted that no distinction was made within the psychotic group and that dysthymics and hysterics are not currently used widely as diagnostic categories. Eysenck postulated that dysthymics (as he called introvert neurotics) differ from hysterics (classified by him as extravert neurotics): Eysenck thought that the two types differed in reactive inhibition in that the former have a slower growth of inhibition than the other type. Perhaps one might think of this as boredom. For the difference between psychotics and normals, Yates emphasized Shakow's work showing consistent impairment in reaction time when an irregular time interval between warning signal and stimulus is used compared to a regular interval. There is still considerable controversy about the interpretation of these findings [Oades, 1982].

Newer research does not use the broad diagnostic groupings of neurotics and psychotics, but realizes that schizophrenia and manic depression are different enough to expect that grouping these two types of mental disorder together will lead to results that cannot be interpreted. Similarly neurotics fall in subgroups differing substantially in their symptomatology. Depressed patients tend to be listless and slow but their motor skills are not fundamentally impaired. Schizophrenics, on the other hand, may have delayed or permanently impaired motor development. Asarnow and Goldstein [1986] have summarized the results of prospective studies of children at risk for schizophrenia. Realizing that at least 85% of schizophrenics do not have schizophrenic parents, other investigators have looked for behavioral warnings in children who later become schizophrenics. In a table compressing results from studies at four life periods (conception to infancy, early childhood, middle childhood, and adolescence), Asarnow and Goldstein [1986] found six studies mentioning abnormal motor functioning in the first period, one study in the second, six studies in the third, and two in the last period. Many studies did not include observations in this area, so they should not be considered as negative instances.

It is less difficult to imagine a relationship between schizophrenics and impaired motor functioning when one realizes that the widely accepted idea of an 'attention deficit' in schizophrenia would imply a reduced ability to concentrate such as is required for many skilled movements, let alone the sustained attention required to acquire a motor skill or proficiency in a sport.

In a recent paper, Manschreck [1983] has reviewed in detail historical evidence for abnormal psychomotor behavior in schizophrenia and relates the impairment to attention deficit [cf. chapter 5 of this book]. He summarized the contributions of Kraepelin, Bleuler, Hughlings, Jackson, Jaspers, Freeman, and psychoanalytic views. Then he discussed more recent investigations from a variety of scientific approaches including neuropharmacologic ones. A German study by Günther and Grüber [1983] used a modification of the Oseretsky test and the motor subtests of the Nebraska-Luria test and found significant differences between 15 drug-free schizophrenics and 15 endogenous and 15 nonendogenous depressed individuals plus 15 normal controls, but no differences between the depressed and the normals.

The Russian scientist Luria combined neurological and psychiatric interests and developed a rather unique system of diagnosing mental abnormalities and their basis in the brain. Charles Golden developed a standard neuropsychological test battery entitled the Nebraska-Luria battery [Golden et al., 1978]. This battery contains a number of motor performance items, similar to, but more varied than the usual neurological tasks. All of the items in the test battery were adapted from Christensen [1975] with modifications needed to establish standard administrative scoring procedures. The battery consists of 282 measures (items) and can be administered in less than 2½ hours. The items fall into the following 10 categories developed from factor analytic studies by Golden and associates:

Motor function: This series of tasks requires the reproduction of simple motor movements with the hands, mouth, and tongue both when a model is provided and from verbal instructions alone. The section also evaluates simple coordinated abilities, motor-spatial organization, complex sequencing of behavior, and the ability to draw.

Acousticomotor (rhythm) functions: These items require the individual to differentiate between sounds with different pitch and different rhythmic relationships. The subject must indicate whether sounds are the same or different and reproduce given pitch or rhythmic relationships played from a tape.

Cutaneous and kinesthetic (tactile) functions: This section evaluates complex cutaneous functions, muscle and joint sensations, and stereognosis. Kinesthetic assessment requires a blindfolded subject to identify the direction of limb movements and reproduce limb position. Cutaneous assessment includes evaluation of threshold localization, stimulus identification, and two-point finger and palm discrimination. The assessment for stereognosis requires a blindfolded subject to identify common objects placed in the palm of the hand.

Visual functions: These tasks assess the integrity of visual-spatial perception, including the identification of objects and pictures, identifying the missing elements in complex geometric configurations (similar to the tasks in Raven's Progressive Matrices), transposing pictures of blocks with no numbers, and showing spatial and directional orientation. Finally, the ability of a subject to perform spatial rotations and transformations is assessed.

Expressive speech: This section includes tasks requiring the articulation of simple speech sounds, familiar and unfamiliar words of varying lengths, and phrases or sentences of varied length and complexity. The test also requires the subject to name and classify objects and to produce narrative descriptions.

Receptive speech: The items here require the patient to discriminate between phonemes, and measure the patient's ability to comprehend simple words, phrases, and sentences. Understanding of complex and inverted grammatical structures is also assessed.

Reading and writing: The subject must break words into their component sounds or letters; integrate sounds or letters into words; write words of varying complexity from dictation; and read letters, words, phrases, and paragraphs.

Arithmetic skills: The subject is required to identify Arabic and Roman numerals, to identify the significance of digit placement, to compare numbers of varying size, and to perform simple arithmetic operations (multiplication, addition, subtraction) and simple algebraic manipulations. The ability to form arithmetic series is also evaluated. Items are presented both orally and visually.

Mnestic processes: The tasks assess an individual's retention and retrieval skills for visual, acoustic, and kinesthetic inputs. Items involve both verbal and nonverbal material. The effects of retroactive and proactive interference are also examined.

Intellectual processes: The final section requires the subject to interpret the themes of pictures, to demonstrate vocabulary skills, to form concepts, to classify objects, to understand analogies, to understand complex arithmetical problems, and to show logical reasoning skills.

The Nebraska-Luria items do not seem to make a significant contribution to the diagnosis of either manic depression or schizophrenia, although subgroups of schizophrenics show motor defects [Golden, pers. commun., 1987].

So it seems that little progress has been made since Yates' 1973 review of abnormalities of motor behavior. What may be needed is a simultaneous attempt to develop a battery of psychomotor tasks suitable for use with normal and mentally ill persons designed for several age groups: adults, adolescents, and younger children. It may also be necessary to take a close look at the Bayley scales for infant testing, the Touwen and Prechtl methods,

Table VI. Spontaneous and drug-induced movement disorders due to dopamine-acetylcholine imbalance

Dopamine excess/acetylcholine deficiency	Dopamine deficiency/acetylcholine excess
Drug-induced	
Tardive dyskinesia	neuroleptic-induced parkinsonism
Tics	neuroleptic-induced dystonia
Chorea	neuroleptic-induced akathisia
Stereotypy	
Spontaneous	
Huntington's chorea	Parkinson's disease
Tourette's syndrome	dystonic musculorum deformans
Sydenham's chorea	
Hemiballism	
Hyperthyroid chorea	
Chorea gravidarum	
Senile chorea	

and the Gesell schedule of examination of infants to see whether a continuity of items can be achieved which would allow predictors of later motor performance from infant items. Günther and Grüber point out that results from a broader battery of motor tasks would contribute to differential diagnosis and provide a theoretical basis for neurochemical research and for therapeutic exercise programs.

Movement Disorders

While Luria's [1973] work is based mainly on treatment of brain-injured soldiers, there are other abnormalities of motor behavior commonly referred to as movement disorders. There are two kinds of movement disorders: *spontaneous* and *drug-induced*. Present thinking makes another distinction which cuts across the previous one: Dopamine deficiency and acetylcholine excess versus the reverse: acetylcholine deficiency and dopamine excess. Table VI lists various disorders classified in the resulting four categories. Current ideas are mostly based on a combination of animal research and clinical experience with patients treated for Parkinson's and other spontaneous disorders as well as treatment of psychiatric patients with psychoactive drugs which led to drug-induced ('iatrogenic') side effects and attempts to alleviate

Table VII. Examples of psychoactive drugs that induce movement disorders

Dopamine agonists (e.g., levodopa, amphetamine, methylphenidate, permoline, bromocriptine, lisuride, pergolide)

Dopamine antagonists (e.g., haloperidol, fluphenazine, chlorpromazine, thioridazine)

Beta-adrenergic enhancing drugs (caffeine, lithium, tricyclic antidepressents, theophyllin, albuterol)

Hormones (e.g., thyroid, estrogen)

MPTP (1-methyl-4-phenyl-1, 2, 3, 6-tetrahydropyridine)

those side affects. Some types of psychoactive drugs are listed in table VII. Actually the situation is discouragingly complicated, because some patients do not suffer the side effects, others only after years of treatment, and others almost immediately. But even worse are the indications that there are not just a few neurotransmitters but perhaps as many as 30–40, and that many receptors are not responding to one transmitter only, but two or more [Stahl, 1986].

Much of the research in this field is of necessity based on trial and error, since the study of biochemical minutiae in the living brain is virtually a closed book. Yet progress is being made and patients are being helped and basic understanding is growing. Eventually all that knowledge will be available to be integrated with our understanding of normal behavior, whether motoric or mental.

Concluding Remarks: New Areas

In recent years attention has been focused on sports and physical fitness activities used for therapeutic purposes. Folkins and Simes [1981] reviewed some of this research. There is another research area which could be brought in contact with the types of investigation discussed in this chapter. Studies of hereditary factors in motor development and performance have been summarized by Malina [1984] and Kovar [1980]. Most of this work has been done in virtual isolation from neuropsychiatric research, but it has a promise of adding fundamentally new insights.

Another neglected area has been the influence of body types and expressive style.

There has been a general decline in interest in body types since the days of Sheldon due to the rather low level of correlation found between personality and body types. There may be more correspondence between body type and specific kinds of sports. For instance, swimmers tend to look somewhat similar to one another as do quarterbacks. The study of expressive movements has fared even less well in recent years. Hardly any new work has been done in this area even though the relevance for sports performance would appear to be obvious. Part of the problem is in the absence of useful, valid, and reliable methods of assessing such variables. In conclusion, this chapter ends with the customary call for more and better research.

References

Asarnow, J.R.; Goldstein, M.J.: Schizophrenia during adolescence and early adulthood: A developmental perspective on risk research. Clin. Psychol. Rev. *6:* 211–235 (1986).

Barrow, H.M.; McGee, R.: A practical approach to measurement in physical education (Lea & Febiger, Philadelphia 1964).

Berger, R.A.: Applied exercise physiology (Lea & Febiger, Philadelphia 1982).

Bayley, N.: Bayley Scales of Infant Development: Manual (Psychological Corporation, New York 1969).

Bolles, R.N.: The three boxes of life, and how to get out of them (Ten Speed Press, Berkeley 1973).

Browne, M.A.; Mahoney, M.J.: Sports psychology. Ann. Rev. Psychol. *35:* 605–626 (1984).

Burke, K.L.: Comparison of psychological androgyny within a sample of female athletes who participate in sports traditionally appropriate and inappropriate for competition by females. Percept. Mot. Skills *63:* 779–782 (1986).

Cerretelli, P.: Exercise and endurance; in Larson, Fitness, health, and work capacity: International Standards for Assessment. (Macmillan, New York 1974).

Christensen, A.L.: Luria's neuropsychological investigation (Spectrum, New York 1975).

Connolly, K.J.; Prechtl, H.F.R.: Maturation and development: Biological and psychological perspectives (Lippincott, Philadelphia 1981).

Csikszentmihaly, M.: Beyond boredom and anxiety. The experience of play in work and games (Jossey-Bass, San Francisco 1975).

Denny-Brown, D.: The general principles of motor integration; in Magoun, Section I: Neurophysiology; vol. 2: Handbook of physiology (Williams & Wilkins, Baltimore 1960).

Eysenck, H.J.: Sex and personality (University of Texas Press, Austin 1976).

Eysenck, H.J.; Wilson, G.: The psychology of sex (Dent, London 1979).

Fish, B.: Biological antecedents of psychosis in children; in Freedman, Biology of the major psychoses (Raven Press, New York 1975).

Fleishman, E.A.: Dimensional analysis of psychomotor abilities. J. exp. Psychol. *48:* 437–454 (1954).

Fleishman, E.A.; Quaintance, M.K.: Taxonomies of human performance: The description of human task (Academic Press, New York 1984).

Foa, U.G.: Convergences in the analysis of the structure of interpersonal behavior. Psychol. Rev. *68:* 341–353 (1961).

Folkins, C.H.; Simes, W.E.: Physical fitness training and mental health. Am. Psychol. *36:* 373–389 (1981).

Freedman, M.B.; Leary, T.; Ossorio, A.G.; Coffey, H.S.: The interpersonal dimensions of personality. J. Personality 20: 143–161 (1951).

Gesell, A.; Amatruda, C.S.: Developmental diagnosis. Normal and abnormal child development (Hoeber, New York 1941).

Ghez, C.: Introduction to the motor systems; in Kandel, Schwartz, Principles of neural science, pp. 429–441 (Elsevier, New York 1985).

Gilbert, D.G.: Marriage and sex: Moving from correlations to dynamic personality by personality interactions – limits of molecular vision; in Modgil, Modgil, Hans Eysenck, consensus and controversy (Falmer Press, London 1986).

Golden, C.J.; Hemmcke, T.; Purisch, A.D.: Diagnostic validity of a standardized neuropsychological battery derived from Luria's neuropsychological tests. J. consult. clin. Psychol. 46: 1258 (1978).

Gough, H.G.; Heilbrun, A.B.: The adjective checklist manual (Consulting Psychologists Press, Palo Alto 1962).

Günther, W.; Grüber, H.: Psychomotorische Störungen bei psychiatrischen Patienten als mögliche Grundlage neuer Ansätze in Differentialdiagnose und Therapie. I. Ergebnisse erster Untersuchungen an depressiven und schizophrenen Kranken. Arch. Psychiat. Nervenkrankh. 233: 187–208 (1983).

Gurewitsch, M.; Oseretsky, N.I.: Zur Methodik der Untersuchung der motorischen Funktionen. Mschr. Psychiat. Neurol. 59: 78–103 (1925).

Holland, J.L.: The psychology of vocational choice (Blaisdell Publishing, Waltham 1966).

Kabanoff, B.: Work and non-work: A review of models, methods, and findings. Psychol. Bull. 88: 60–71 (1980).

Kabanoff, B.; O'Brien, G.E.: Work and leisure: A task attributes analysis. J. appl. Psychol. 65: 596–609 (1980).

Kandel, E.R.; Schwartz, J.H.: Principles of neural science, 2nd ed. (Elsevier, New York 1981).

Kirkcaldy, B.D.: Personality and sex differences related to positions in team sports. Int. J. Sport Psychol. 13: 141–153 (1982).

Kirkcaldy, B.D.: The value of traits in sport; in Kirkcaldy, Individual differences in movement (MTP, Boston 1985).

Knapp, B.: Skill in sport. The attainment of proficiency (Routledge & Kegan Paul, London 1963).

Kovar, R.: Human variation in motor abilities and its genetic analysis (Faculty of Physical Education and Sports; Charles University, Prague 1980).

Kretchmer, E.: Physique and character (Kegan Paul, London 1936).

Larson, L.A.: Fitness, health and work capacity: International standards for assessment. Int. Comm. for the Standardization of Physical Fitness Tests (Macmillan, New York 1974).

Laski, M.: Ecstacy: A study of some secular and religious experiences (Cresset Press, London 1961).

Leary, T.: Interpersonal diagnosis of personality (Ronald Press, New York 1957).

Lockwood, R.J.; Larkind, D.; Wann, J.: Specific motor disabilities; in Lockwood, Physical education and disability (in press, 1988).

Lorr, M.; Bishop, P.F.; McNair, D.M.: Interpersonal types among psychiatric patients. J. abnorm. Psychol. 70: 468–471 (1955).

Lorr, M.; McNair, D.M.: An interpersonal behavior circle. J. abnorm. soc. Psychol. 67: 68–75 (1965a).

Lorr, M.; McNair, D.M.: Expansion of the interpersonal behavior circle. J. Pers. soc. Psychol. *2:* 823–830 (1965b).

Lorr, M.; Suziekelis, A.: Modes of interpersonal behavior. Br. J. soc. clin. Psychol. *8:* 124–132 (1969).

Luria, A.R.: The working brain: An introduction to neuropsychology (Basic Books, New York 1973).

Magoun, H.W.: Section I: Neurophysiology; vol. 2: Handbook of physiology (Williams & Wilkins, Baltimore 1960).

Maier, R.A.; Lavrakas, P.J.: Some personality correlates of attitudes about sports. Int. J. Sport Psychol. *12:* 19–22 (1981).

Malina, R.M.: Genetics of motor development and performance; in Malina, Bouchard, The 1984 Olympic Scientific Congress Proceeding (Human Kinetics Publishers, Champaign 1984).

Malpass, L.F.: Motor proficiency in institutionalized and non-institutionalized retarded children and normal children. Am. J. ment. Defic. *64:* 1012–1015 (1960).

Manschreck, T.: Psychopathology of motor behavior in schizophrenia; in Mahler, Mahler, Progress in experimental personality research, vol. 12 (Academic Press, New York 1983).

Mathews, D.K.: Measurement in physical education (Saunders, Philadelphia 1973).

McKechnie, G.E.: A study of environmental life styles; unpubl. diss. (University of California, Berkeley 1972).

McKechnie, G.E.: The psychological structure of leisure: Past behavior J. Leisure Res. *6:* 27–45 (1974).

McKernon, J.G.: The relationship between intelligence and motor proficiency in the intellectually gifted child; unpubl. diss. (University of Denver, Denver 1956).

Morehouse, I.E.; Rasch, P.I.: Sports medicine for trainers, 2nd ed. (Saunders, Philadelphia 1964).

Oades, R.D.: Attention and schizophrenia, neurobiological bases (Pitman Advanced Publishing Program, London 1982).

Oseretsky, N.I.: Zur Methodik der Untersuchung der motorischen Komponenten. Z. angew. Psychol. *32:* 257–293 (1929).

Oseretsky, N.I.: Psychomotorik: Methoden zur Untersuchung der Motorik. Beih. Psychol. *57* (1931).

Pestonje, D.M.; Singh, R.B.; Singh, A.P.; Singh, U.B.: Personality and physical abilities: An empirical investigation. Int. J. Sport Psychol. *12:* 39–51 (1981).

Ruch, T.C.; Patton, H.O.: Physiology and biophysics: The brain and neural function (Saunders, Philadelphia 1974).

Schaefer, E.S.: A configural analysis of children's reports of parental behavior. J. consult. Psychol. *29:* 552–557 (1966).

Schulz, W.C.: FIRO: A three-dimensional theory of interpersonal behavior (Rinehart, New York 1958).

Schulz, W.C.: FIRO-B (Consulting Psychologists Press, Palo Alto 1967).

Smyth, M.H.; Wing, A.M.: The psychology of human movement (Academic Press, New York 1984).

Spranger, E.: Lebensformen; 2nd ed. (Niemeyer, Halle 1921).

Stahl, S.M.: Neuropharmacology of movement disorders: Comparison of spontaneous and drug-induced movement disorders; in Shah, Donald, Movement disorders (Plenum Medical, New York 1986).

Stern, G.G.; Stein, M.I.; Bloom, B.S.: Methods in personality assessment (Free Press, Glencoe 1986).

Straub, W.F.: Sensation seeking among high- and low-risk male athletes. J. Sport Psychol. *4:* 246–253 (1982).

Sullivan, H.S.: The interpersonal theory of psychiatry (Norton, New York 1953).

Thams, P.F.: A factor analysis of the Lincoln-Oseretsky Motor Development Scale; unpubl. diss. (University of Michigan, Ann Arbor 1955).

Touwen, B.C.L.; Prechtl, H.F.R.: The neurological examination of the child with minor neurological dysfunction (Lippincott, Philadelphia 1970).

Van Der Lugt, M.J.A.: Psychomotor test series for children for the measurement of manual ability (New York University, New York 1949).

Vandenberg, S.G.: Factor analytic studies of the Lincoln-Oseretsky test of motor proficiency. Percept. Mot. Skills *19:* 23–41 (1964).

Wiggins, J.S.: Personality and prediction: Principles of personality assessment (Addison-Wesley, Reading 1973).

Wilson, G.: Personality, sexual behavior and marital satisfaction; in Modgil, Modgil, Hans Eysenck, consensus and controversy (Falmer Press, London 1986).

Wing, A.M.: Disorders of movement; in Smyth, Wing, The psychology of human movement, pp. 269–296 (Academic Press, New York 1984).

Wulfeck, W.H.: Motor function in the mentally disordered. Psychol. Rec. *4:* 271–323 (1941).

Yarmolenko, A.: The motor sphere of school-age children. J. genet. Psychol. *4:* 298–316 (1933).

Yates, A.J.: Abnormalities of psychomotor function; in Eysenck, Handbook of abnormal psychology (Knapp, San Diego 1973).

Zuckerman, M.: Sensation seeking. Beyond the optimal level of arousal (Erlbaum, Hillsdale 1979).

Steven G. Vandenberg, PhD, Institute for Behavioral Genetics, University of Colorado, Boulder, CO 80309–0447 (USA)

Kirkcaldy B (ed): Normalities and Abnormalities in Human Movement.
Med Sport Sci. Basel, Karger, 1989, vol 29, pp 36–57

A Multiple-Representations' Approach to Mental Practice of Motor Skills[1]

Herbert Heuer

Fachbereich Psychologie der Philipps-Universität Marburg, FRG

The importance of understanding mental practice of motor skills is obvious from an applied point of view. This mode of practice is familiar in the field of physical education, and it is likely to be useful in the rehabilitation of motor disorders caused by damage to the central nervous system [Guenther, 1980]. In fact, the majority of studies on mental practice has been conducted to explore particular applications. There are numerous experiments which examine the effects of mental practice on certain skills in certain populations. Although such a strategy of research may provide quick answers to questions of current practical relevance, it also makes the field look somewhat scattered and disconnected. As seems often to be the case with applied research, the studies are scarcely linked to each other and contribute negligibly to the development of integrative theories [Heuer, 1988]. Beyond each particular result there are only a few tentative generalizations that can be made, and these generally appear more like descriptions of the outcome of some kind of opinion poll than as stringent generalizations covering the available data [e.g. Thomas, 1978, pp. 147–148; Volkamer, 1972].

With respect to the mechanisms of mental practice effects two dominant hypotheses have emerged which will be discussed and evaluated in the course of this chapter. In addition to these two hypotheses several more have been proposed that occasionally leave a somewhat strange impression. Moreover, mental practice effects are closely associated with *ideomotor phenomena* which sometimes have been invoked to explain paranormal phenomena [Richter, 1954]. Thus by theorizing about mental practice one is endangered

---

[1] This chapter is based on a paper entitled 'Wie wirkt mentale Übung?' which appeared in Psychologische Rundschau, *36:* 191–200 (1985).

into trespassing in the irrational sphere. This danger probably results from the need to explain how the *mental* affects the *physical* domain. Fortunately, however, what distinguishes mental practice effects from psychokinetics and other paranormal phenomena is that mental practice and subsequent execution of the skill are related to one and the same brain.

During recent years a certain change can be observed in the general orientation of cognitive psychology which brings mental practice more into the core area of theoretical interest. While cognitive psychology started as the study of the 'fate of the stimulus', it became increasingly recognized that cognition is not a purpose in itself but rather has to serve action. 'Stimulus orientation' of research is thus supplemented by 'action orientation' [Heuer and Prinz, 1987]. From this perspective, mental practice becomes an exemplary field for the study of the relation between cognitive processes and motor control. The core question is how the apparently disparate areas of mental and physical phenomena are related to each other. The basic answer, of course, is that these classes of phenomena are not really disparate, but rather that motor control is to some extent a cognitive process, so that there is nothing mysterious about the effects of mental practice.

This chapter is intended as an evaluative and selective review of the major hypotheses. As it turns out, these hypotheses fit neatly within a multiple representations' framework of skilled movements. Such a framework does not only permit a better understanding of mental practice effects, but also brings mental practice into closer contact with the general field of motor control and learning, as well as with imagery research. Due to this emphasis of the chapter, I do not claim completeness in the coverage of the relevant literature. For readers interested in a rather complete overview, several review papers are available [Richardson, 1967a, b; Corbin, 1972; Feltz and Landers, 1983].

What Is Mental Practice?

Rather than providing a definition, this question shall be answered by means of a classical study, that of Vandell et al. [1943]. (Needs for definitions are dealt with satisfactorily by Volkamer [1972] or Ungerer [1977, p. 62].) On the one hand, this study illustrates the phenomenon and, on the other, the experimental design on which almost all of the later experiments are based.

Vandell and colleagues tested dart-throwing and the basketball free-shot in three experiments with subjects of various age ranges. Three groups of subjects took part in each experiment; each performed a pretest (25 or

Table I. Percentage improvement in the three experiments of Vandell et al. [1943]

Experiment	Group		
	no practice	physical practice	mental practice
I Dart-throwing	− 2	+ 7	+ 4
II Basketball free-shot	+ 2	+ 41	+ 43
III Dart-throwing	0	+ 23	+ 22

35 throws) on the 1st day and a similar posttest on the 20th day. During the interval between pretest and posttest there were no contacts between the no-practice control group and the experimenter, whereas the physical-practice control group performed 25 or 35 throws daily – just as on the test days. The subjects assigned to the mental-practice experimental group participated in a daily session of 15 or 30 min. The instructions for these sessions required the subjects to imagine themselves while performing the skill to be acquired. This instruction can be considered the standard instruction for mental practice; the subjects' actual responses to this instruction, however, are less clear.

The findings of Vandell et al. [1943] are shown in table I: mental practice proved to be just as effective as physical practice. This result is atypical, however. In most studies the improvement of the mental-practice group lies between that of the no-practice control group and the physical-practice control group. With mixed forms of physical and mental practice, the improvement of the physical-practice group is sometimes exceeded [e.g. Ulich, 1967; Willimczik et al., 1976], but a larger improvement through mental practice alone compared to physical practice is rarely found [e.g. Minas, 1978, 1980].

How Can Mental-Practice Effects Be Explained?

The various hypotheses advanced in the literature can be classified into specific, unspecific and 'strange' ones. The latter two categories of hypotheses shall be touched only briefly, the first one will be dealt with in more detail.

The category of strange hypotheses may be illustrated by an example which has recently been described at least twice, apparently independent of each other [Mendoza and Wichman, 1978; Zecker, 1982]. According to this hypothesis, mental practice constitutes a particular variety of *imitation*. If a subject imagines himself/herself performing a motor pattern, this can be considered as being equivalent to observing a model. If, in addition, the performance of the imagined activity is successful, then what could be referred to as 'self-imitation', is vicariously [Mendoza and Wichman, 1978], or secondarily [Zecker, 1982] reinforced. This hypothesis obviously tries to explain something that requires no explanation: at some time or other the subject performs the imagined motor skill. No explanation is given, however, for the observation that performance improves with mental practice.

Unspecific hypotheses are those that attribute the effects of mental practice to a relatively unspecific increase in motivation or *effort*. It is quite obvious that such effects can show up in all studies of mental practice. From a theoretical point of view, however, unspecific effects of mental practice are of little interest. It is mainly a problem of the experimental design to adequately control for them and to bring the more interesting specific effects into the foreground.

Hidden unspecific effects are likely to exist in earlier studies of mental practice, such as that of Vandell et al., where the no-practice control group was not in contact with the experimenter during the practice periods of the other groups which lasted several days. Recent studies generally avoid this obvious source of a *Hawthorne* effect by further making the no-practice control group perform defined experimental activities. It is not possible, however, to rule out with certainty unspecific effects through such methodological refinements.

There are at least two ways to eliminate unspecific effects more reliably. First, a control group analogous to the *placebo* group in pharmacopsychological experiments could be introduced: subjects perform activities which have no practice effect on the skill under study; they are convinced, however, that these activities improve their performance. The second method requires at least two very similar tasks to be tested, only one of which is being practiced. Such an approach implies that unspecific effects of mental practice should appear in both tasks, in contrast to specific effects, which predict limitation to one task. From my knowledge, the first approach has not been pursued so far, the second one just once [MacKay, 1981].

Specific Effects of Mental Practice

Taking strict formal criteria into account, specific effects of mental practice beyond possible unspecific effects have hardly been substantiated so far. There are plausible reasons to believe, however, that the effects of mental practice are to a large extent of a specific nature. In the following, for instance, findings are dealt with which imply that mental practice has different effects on different types of tasks. These differences can easily be understood as a result of specific processes of learning, but hardly as a result of different degrees of sensitivity of various tasks to differences in the subjects' motivation or effort.

As mentioned above, two major hypotheses have emerged over the years to explain the specific effects of mental practice. These hypotheses seem to be based on the following implicit assumptions: (1) mental practice of cognitive skills is more or less natural; (2) the same is true for physical practice of motor skills, and (3) mental practice of motor skills, however, presents a puzzle. Under these premises the problem of mental practice of motor skills can be regarded as basically solved if it can be reduced to one of the two cases described first. That is exactly what both major hypotheses aim at:

(1) According to the *cognitive hypothesis*, mental practice effects are restricted to the cognitive components of motor skills. Motor skills are essentially treated as cognitive skills.

(2) According to the *ideomotor* or *psychoneuromuscular hypothesis*, mental practice comprises a physical component that causes its effects. Here mental practice is essentially treated as physical practice.

In order to put the two hypotheses in a conceptual framework it is useful to ask in which way a movement can be described and, at the same time, how it can be learned. The answer to this question is likely to differ depending on whether open or closed skills [Poulton, 1957] are considered. Since the majority of studies of mental practice deal with closed skills which need not be adapted to a varying environment, such restrictions will be observed here, too.

A Multiple-Representations Framework for Motor-Skills Learning

A closed skill such as a basketball free-shot can obviously be described in different ways. There are at least four:

(1) The *motor description* specifies the spatiotemporal pattern of efferent commands.

(2) The *kinesthetic description* specifies the kinesthetic accompaniments of the motor pattern, that is, how it 'feels'.

(3) The *visuospatial description* specifies spatiotemporal characteristics of the seen movement. In imagining a movement, it may correspond to an

'external perspective', that of an observer, whereas the kinesthetic description necessarily corresponds to an 'internal perspective', that of an actor
[Epstein, 1980].

(4) Finally, a *symbolic* or *verbal description* is to be mentioned.

It may be ignored here that for a motor pattern achieving a certain result
like throwing, any of these various descriptions may not be unique since a
particular result can usually be achieved using different motor patterns, as
demonstrated in throwing by Stimpel [1933]. Rather the descriptions should
refer to classes of motor patterns with certain characteristics, the result being
invariant for the members of the class.

The fact that motor patterns can be described in different ways implies
the possibility that they might also be learned in different ways. Once this
latter possibility is considered, the four kinds of descriptions change their
formal status. No longer are they merely different aspects of a movement
which can be used for description, but rather they acquire something which is
sometimes referred to as 'psychological reality'. It is postulated that it is
possible to develop *internal representations* of a motor pattern which correspond to these descriptions. The question as to what extent such representations are actually used in performing different tasks is of an experimental
nature.

For the present purpose it is only important that, in principle, all four
kinds of internal representations of a motor pattern can be present; it is not
of importance, however, under what conditions they are actually generated.
The potential existence of pure *motor* representations, for example, follows
from the finding that it is possible to learn movements even in the absence of
any sensory information [e.g. Taub et al., 1975]. The potential existence of
kinesthetic representations is indicated by the finding that movements can be
learned more precisely if there is kinesthetic feedback, and that, if kinesthetic
feedback is present, other features of a movement seem to be learned than
when it is not present [Heuer, 1983, pp. 77–78]. The importance of *visuospatial* representations and *symbolic* representations, finally, becomes evident
from experiments in which the interference between symbolic or visuospatial
tasks and motor performance is studied. Clear results are available in particular for spatial imagery [Heuer and Wing, 1984], whereas corresponding
studies using verbal tasks have been conducted less frequently [e.g. Adams,
1981].

The four kinds of representations discussed above are certainly not the
only ones that can exist. It may well be that separate representations can be
found for almost any descriptive characteristic of a motor pattern. Thus, the

four kinds of representations also serve an illustrative purpose, and the considerations that follow with respect to these representations can be generalized to others. A multiple-representations' framework is open with respect to the specific kinds of representations included. What is essential in applying this framework to mental practice phenomena is evident in two questions which are asked with respect to each representation, and here I shall consider these questions with respect to the four representations described:

(1) What is the link between a particular representation and performance?

(2) How accessible is a particular representation for cognitive manipulations?

Representations and Performance

It is quite obvious that, having learned a motor representation of a movement, the movement can actually be performed. The ability to drive the peripheral machinery of muscles and bones is more or less the central feature of a motor representation. The situation is quite different, however, if kinesthetic, visuospatial or symbolic representations are considered. These representations do not by themselves include the motor commands indispensable to performance. Whereas there is still a rather close relationship between kinesthesia and efferent commands – efferent commands, for instance, seem to contribute to the perception of movements [e.g. Lashley, 1917; Kelso, 1977] – the other representations seem to scarcely exhibit any relation to the motor commands. Activity of the central nervous system during visual perception of a movement or its visual imagination, for instance, is likely to be entirely different from the activity involved in execution of that movement. What are the benefits of learning such representations for skilled performance?

There is a simple answer to this question: learning symbolic, visuospatial or kinesthetic representations is advantageous if the relation between those representations and the corresponding motor commands is known; i.e. if they can be transformed into the corresponding *motor commands*. The distinction between known and unknown relations will appear repeatedly in the following. It is certain to be a rather unsatisfactory distinction since it does not indicate how a transformation is possible between representations which, initially, are entirely different.

For the present purpose, detailed assumptions about the processes involved in transformations between representations are not needed. Rather it is sufficient to state that sometimes non-motor representations can be transformed into motor representations, whereas on other occasions they cannot. Nonetheless, it might be helpful in understanding the relations between different kinds of representations and actual performance to provide some sketch of how transformations could be achieved in principle. One way of solving the transformation problem would be to store correlations.

The concept of 'correlation storage' originates from Hein and Held [1962] and refers to flexible relations between visual information and efferent output. It is in fact similar to the notion of a 'recall schema' advanced by Schmidt [1975]. The basic assumption is that the relations between visual input and efferent commands (or between any other two kinds of signals) are learned by way of covariations, that is, by experiencing the visual consequences of certain motor commands. The correlation storage is essentially a reference table assigning particular motor commands to visual consequences and vice versa. It is not difficult to conceive how such transformation tables (or probably rules rather than tables) could be set up which relate any two modalities to each other, e.g. the kinesthetic feedback usually associated with certain visual information about a moving limb.

The correlation store as conceived by Hein and Held [1962] is concerned with actual sensory information or motor commands. The concept can, however, easily be generalized to cover relations between internal representations. It might even be the same transformation rules that are applied for example in reaching to an actually seen target and to a target whose spatial location is remembered; the sensory input might just be replaced by the visuospatial representation of the target.

Correlation theories for transformations between different kinds of representations imply that the relations have to be learned and can be changed under appropriate conditions. The ability to transform one representation into another thus does critically depend on learning. There may be visuospatial representations of movement patterns for which transformation rules do exist, while for others they do not exist. Thus, correlation theories lead one to expect that there are cases in which transformations are possible, whereas in others they are impossible. They do not, of course, exclude the possibility that processes other than the use of stored correlations may be involved in transformations, e.g. taking advantage of identical temporal characteristics of different representations [Prinz, 1985].

Representations and Cognitive Manipulations

While motor representations have a tight linkage to actual performance, it is hard to see how they could be subjected to cognitive manipulations. For example, it is an easy task to imagine how one performs a giant swing at the high bar. One can visualize one's body rotating around the bar, but our introspection does not appear to reveal anything about the motor commands necessary for performing this feat. Thus it seems to be possible to establish a visuospatial representation by purely cognitive means, but not a motor representation. As I shall argue below, however, some cognitive manipulations of motor representations might be possible although we do not experience anything 'motor'.

Cognitive manipulations of kinesthetic representations appear to be possible to some extent. We can imagine the feel of a certain motor pattern and we can manipulate it in that we imagine a somewhat different feel. At least movement imagination with a clearly kinesthetic quality is possible, although it is not fully clear as to what extent such imaginations can go beyond what we have actually experienced kinesthetically.

Finally, symbolic and visuospatial representations are easily accessible to purely cognitive manipulations. The respective descriptions can be communicated directly, and they can be instructed and learned without the corresponding movement ever having been performed. There is no difficulty in generating a visual image of ourselves performing a particular motor pattern, or in generating a sequence of symbols that refer to a particular sequence of movements.

Putting the answers to the two fundamental questions of a multiple-representations' approach to mental practice together, there appears to be a trade-off between the accessibility of a representation to cognitive manipulations and the tightness of its links to actual performance. Motor and kinesthetic representations have a direct or moderately direct link to performance, but cognitive manipulation is hardly possible, or only within limits. Conversely, symbolic or visuospatial representations only display an indirect link to performance via additional transformation rules, but they can easily be manipulated.

The Cognitive Hypothesis

According to the cognitive hypothesis, mental practice is the manipulation of those representations that are easily accessible, namely symbolic or visuospatial ones. Hence, mental practice is supposed to be mediated by changes of those representations that are somewhat remote from actual performance and linked to it only via additional *transformation rules*.

From the cognitive hypothesis it follows directly that with different tasks, mental practice should be effective in varying degrees. Intuitively, tasks may be classified as 'rather cognitive' or 'rather motor'. Finding one's way through a maze, for instance, is a rather cognitive task, but balancing on a stabilometer or performing a giant swing on the high bar are rather motor.

The distinction between cognitive and motor tasks can be defined more clearly conceptually by referring to the various kinds of representations. Tasks for which the relations between symbolic and visuospatial representations on the one hand and motor representations on the other are known from the onset, are rather cognitive. In this case, acquired symbolic or visuospatial representations can be transformed into motor commands immediately, allowing for execution of the corresponding motor pattern.

If the relations are unknown, however, acquiring symbolic or visuospatial representations is not particularly helpful, and may even be useless with respect to performance. For these 'motor' tasks, kinesthetic and/or motor representations are to be acquired directly. It is clear, that, according to the cognitive hypothesis, a greater effect of mental practice is expected with rather 'cognitive' tasks than with rather 'motor' ones. This is one of the best substantiated results [Feltz and Landers, 1983] which is briefly illustrated in the following study.

Ryan and Simons [1981] compared the effects of mental practice on maze performance and balancing on a stabilometer. (The stabilometer is a platform, mounted on a horizontal axis, on which the subject is required to stand.) The experiment included the three traditional groups who – between pre- and posttest – practiced mentally or physically for eight trials or played 'scrabble' for the same period. As shown in figure 1, the improvement achieved by the mental-practice group lies invariably intermediate to those of both control groups. In the case of maze-learning the improvement is larger than in the no-practice group, but it does not differ significantly from that of the physical-practice group. As for acquiring the skill of balancing, however, the improvement is smaller than after physical practice and does not differ significantly from that of the no-practice control group.

The cognitive hypothesis helps to understand why mental practice is inferior to physical practice in most cases, whilst being superior on other occasions [e.g. Minas, 1978, 1980]. The general inferiority is due to the practice effects being restricted to symbolic or visuospatial representations. These may become perfect over the course of practice, but there is no improvement in transforming these representations into actual motor commands as occurs in physical practice. Consequently, to the extent that the

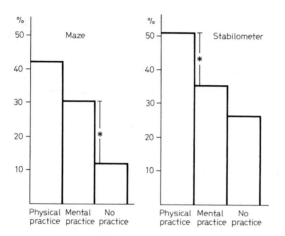

Fig. 1. Effect of mental practice on maze performance and balancing on a stabilometer [from Ryan and Simons, 1981].

transformation rules are less than perfect (or less accurate than after physical practice), performance will be less than perfect. Mental practice in this case induces only part of those changes that are induced by physical practice.

The situation is different when the transformation rules are already perfect when practice commences. In this case any change of the symbolic or visuospatial representation will show up as a corresponding change in performance. In fact, all that there is to learn can be learned on the level of these representations. But learning can be impaired if a second task is to be performed simultaneously [e.g. Nissen and Bullemer, 1987]. It seems that performing the movements to be learned can impair learning in the same manner as any other secondary task does. Minas [1980], for example, had her subjects learn to hop through a certain sequence of squares marked on the floor. What has to be learned in this task appears to be the sequence of squares rather than hopping through a known sequence. Hopping itself seems to distract from learning the sequence. Thus, whenever the rules for transforming symbolic or visuospatial representations into motor commands are well established at the start of practice, there is a chance that mental practice will be superior to physical practice, since actually performing the movement has the potential of impairing the learning of the symbolic or visuospatial representations.

There is little doubt about the validity of the cognitive hypothesis. However, it is doubtful whether this hypothesis is suitable for explaining *all* the effects of mental practice, or whether there remains, so to speak, a *'noncognitive remnant'* which cannot be attributed to learning symbolic or visuospatial representations of motor patterns.

There is probably no argument that conclusively demonstrates the existence of a 'noncognitive remnant', but some arguments can be advanced which make its existence plausible. Mental practice, for instance, affects tasks where the effect is difficult to explain by means of the cognitive hypothesis. An example of such a task is 'balancing on the stabilometer'. It is true that, according to Ryan and Simons [1981], the improvement through mental practice is not significantly larger than that of the no-practice control group, but Ryan and Simons [1982] report a difference of that kind if the subjects are instructed to concentrate on visuospatial and kinesthetic imagery during the periods of mental practice. Similarly, the effects of mental practice on the accuracy of throwing, i.e. the accuracy of very brief ballistic movements, which have been described frequently, are inadequately explained by learning of symbolic or visuospatial representations.

In the following it is assumed that the effects of mental practice cannot be fully explained by the cognitive hypothesis. This assumption, however, cannot be regarded as definitively substantiated. Thus the remainder of this chapter might refer to a non-existent phenomenon. First the question is raised whether the traditional ideomotor hypothesis is appropriate for explaining the 'noncognitive remnant'; the answer to this question will be negative. Subsequently, a modification of the ideomotor hypothesis will be outlined according to which part of mental practice effects is due to cognitive manipulations of motor representations.

The Ideomotor Hypothesis

The basic feature of the ideomotor hypothesis is the assumption of a tight link between the imagination of a movement and its execution. The tight link is known as the ideomotor principle according to which any imagination of a movement is accompanied by a tendency towards its realization [Prinz, 1985]. This principle is obviously attractive in theoretical terms. The gap between the phenomenal world of intentions and imaginations and the physical world of movements is bridged in a very simple way. Accordingly, the principle was heavily burdened from a theoretical point of view, not only with the explanation of mental practice, but also with the explanation of mass phenomena and thought-reading. These theoretical excesses are no longer in a reasonable relation to the experimental foundation of the principle [Richter, 1954, 1957].

The ideomotor hypothesis of mental practice refers predominantly to the work of Jacobson in the early thirties [review paper: Jacobson, 1932]. These studies were not aimed at examining the ideomotor principle, nor at explaining mental practice, but at supporting peripheralistic theories of mental activity. Jacobson showed that the imagination of a certain movement, e.g. flexing an arm, leads to increased myoelectric activity coupled with minimal movement. This peripheral effect is specific to the arm involved in the imagination, and is found only with kinesthetic but not visuospatial imagery. [For a comprehensive review of studies on peripheral effects of imagery, see McGuigan, 1978.]

According to the ideomotor hypothesis, the main burden of explaining the effects of mental practice rests with the minimal peripheral effects of movement imaginations. These peripheral effects serve to conceptually make mental practice basically equivalent to physical practice. In fact, during mental practice increased task-related myoelectric activity can be detected in the respective limb [Wehner et al. 1984]; the intensity of this activity, however, does not yield a monotonic relation to the success of mental practice [Ulich, 1967] – and that presents a problem for the hypothesis. A second difficulty is the fact that images of movements do not necessarily involve peripheral side effects [Richter, 1957].

The ideomotor hypothesis of mental practice becomes untenable if one asks in which way the peripheral side effects of imaginations of movements may lead to improvement. The literature gives two different answers to this question.

The first answer is a simple statement maintaining that the peripheral side effects 'transfer' to the actual performance of the motor pattern [e.g. Wrisberg and Ragsdale, 1979]. This answer seems to imply that sensorimotor learning occurs in the muscles. The only process that might take place in the muscles, however, is an increase in muscular strength, and there is general consensus that mental practice is inappropriate for increasing muscle strength [Corbin, 1972; Feltz and Landers, 1983].

The second and more frequently mentioned answer to the question about the benefits of the peripheral side effects of *movement imagery* refers to the evaluation of kinesthetic feedback thus generated. This hypothesis deserves closer scrutiny. First, it is necessary to distinguish between two distinct meanings of 'feedback' in the motor-learning domain. It can be used to designate an error signal, e.g. in studies of knowledge of results; such error information is of value for improving performance. It is, however, also used to designate signals that convey information about the state of a certain object such as a limb. Kinesthetic feedback is a set of signals of the latter kind.

What is the potential use of kinesthetic feedback for learning? Its only possible use is in checking the correctness of the transformation of a kinesthetic representation into motor commands. Kinesthetic feedback can be compared with the reference – the kinesthetic representation – and errors can be used to adjust the transformation rules. It cannot, however, be used to improve the transformation rules which lead from symbolic or visuospatial representations to kinesthetic ones. Thus, the usefulness of kinesthetic feedback for learning is rather restricted when no other information about what has to be learned is available.

More importantly, kinesthetic feedback during movement imagery shares only a remote resemblance to that during movement execution. Some receptors like those in the joints may barely be involved during imagery, while other receptors like muscle spindles and tendon organs may be active, but with strongly attenuated intensities. At best, the temporal pattern of their activity might be similar to the temporal pattern during performance. As a result, there will always be a mismatch between kinesthetic feedback during movement imagery and an internal reference. It is difficult to see how any improvement of motor performance could arise under such conditions. In conclusion, it is highly improbable that the peripheral side effects of movement imagery play a role in mental practice effects.

The Programming Hypothesis

In this section, a modification of the ideomotor hypothesis shall be outlined which seems more appropriate for explaining the 'noncognitive remnant' of the effects of mental practice. The basic idea is not to assume the peripheral side effects of imaginations of movements to be essential for the effects of mental practice, but rather the central process implicated by them. The improvement of performance by repetitions of the central process can be attributed to two factors: (a) the practicing effect of repetitions themselves; this corresponds to Thorndike's *law of exercise*, and (b) the correction of the central process based on internal feedback and some reference.

The central process indicated by the peripheral side effects of movement imagery can be referred to as programming, and the modification of the ideomotor hypothesis can accordingly be labelled, the programming hypothesis. According to this hypothesis, imaginations of movements involve providing the appropriate motor commands which, however, are not transferred to the periphery of the body. The central processes during imagination of a movement should be largely identical with those found during performance. (This hypothesis does not imply the reverse, namely that any programming of a movement involves its imagination.)

There is little experimental evidence supporting the hypothesis that imaginations of a movement are accompanied by programming it. The strongest piece of evidence was presented by Roland et al. [1980] who measured the degree of activation of different cortical areas in terms of oxygen supply. When performing a certain sequence of finger movements, an increased activity was mainly found in the primary sensorimotor cortex with its monosynaptic connections to the motoneurons and in the supplementary motor area. If the subjects were instructed to imagine the same sequence of finger movements, increased activity was found only in the supplementary motor area, but no longer in the primary sensorimotor areas. Thus, the cortical areas activated during imagination of a movement sequence seem to be a subset of those areas that are activated during performance, with the difference predominantly including those areas which exhibit the most direct connections to the periphery of the body.

One aspect of the programming hypothesis, that becomes apparent in the study of Roland et al. [1980], will be emphasized. In discussing the cognitive hypothesis, the importance of knowing the rules for transforming different representations of a movement into motor commands was stressed. Similarly, one might inquire about the importance of knowing the relation between kinesthetic representations and motor commands with regard to the programming hypothesis. This question implicitly assumes that imaginations of movements are 'attenuated or faint kinesthetic perceptions' [Weimer, 1977], since it is only in this case that the question arises. Therefore it is irrelevant to the programming hypothesis since, according to this hypothesis, imaginations of movements are not 'faint perceptions', but additionally or solely movements with blocked final pathways. In this sense the imagination of a movement *is* a movement; the difference between a movement and the imagination of a movement essentially lies in the fact that in the first, but not in the second case, the centrally generated commands are transmitted to the periphery of the body [MacKay, 1982].

If the assumption that imagining a movement is accompanied by its programming is valid, how can improved performance be explained? One possibility is that the practicing effect of imaginations of movements can simply be attributed to the repeated programming involved. Consequently, the particular problem of mental practice is reduced to the more general problem of how repeated performance of a movement can lead to improvement. The particularity of mental practice arises whilst the motor pattern is not repeated on all levels of control but only in its essential central components which, however, should be basic to any improvement.

Reducing the effect of mental practice to a general law of exercise may seem questionable since, at least in the field of sensorimotor skills, the applicability of this law has not generally been accepted. It is obvious that certain characteristics of movement cannot be acquired without knowledge of results. At least in classical studies characteristics had to be learned about which the subjects had not received any information except by knowledge of results [Heuer, 1983, pp. 65–68]. Regarding those characteristics, however, for which the information contained in knowledge of results is irrelevant, it should be possible to improve performance simply by repetition. If, for example, it is postulated that repeated performance or programming of a motor pattern leads to facilitation of neuronal connections, then an increase in speed and probably a decrease of variability is to be expected [MacKay, 1982]. This, of course, will only be manifested as improvement if the performance measure comprises speed and/or variability.

A second possible answer to the question as to how repeated programming of a motor pattern might result in an improvement of performance is based on the assumption of *internal knowledge of results* which gives rise to corrections of the program. This is certain to be a rather speculative assumption on which I should like to comment.

As far as I know, the assumption of internal knowledge of results was first exposed in the theory of Adams [1971]. Thereafter it was adopted by Schmidt [1975] and included in his schema theory, avoiding the logical error implicit in Adam's theory. This assumption presumes: (1) The existence of at least two representations of the movement, e.g. a motor and a kinesthetic one (the assumption of at least two representations is an essential ingredient of the multiple representations' framework). (2) A possible dissociation of both representations which is likely to happen particularly in the case of fast ballistic movements; as for such movements the time available during the movement itself is insufficient for adjusting the motor program to the kinesthetic representation. Only after the movement has ceased can a deviation be detected and utilized for a correction of the motor representation, which will show up in the following movement. An everyday example that may be interpreted in terms of internal knowledge of results occurs with throwing: sometimes a miss is already noticed when the object thrown has barely left the hand.

Internal knowledge of results, as postulated by Adams [1971] and Schmidt [1975] with respect to real movements can also be postulated with respect to imagined and programmed movements, at least if they are brief and ballistic. It should be noted that the hypothesis of internal knowledge of results contributing to mental practice effects is not very different from the hypothesis that the peripheral side effects of movement imagery make some contribution. In both cases some kind of feedback has to be compared with an internal reference such as a kinesthetic representation, and the error signal is used to improve the motor representation or the rules for transforming a kinesthetic representation into motor commands. The major difference between the two hypotheses is that whereas the limitations of the peripheral feedback during movement imagery are known about, we have no idea about the internal processes leading to internal knowledge of results. Although there is no convincing evidence on the role of internal knowledge of results being involved in mental practice effects, data are available which indicate that the hypothesis should not be discarded prematurely.

An initial problem for which data are available concerns the transferability of the concept of internal knowledge of results from overt to imagined movements. Supposing that the effect of mental practice is – at least partially – due to an evaluation of internal knowledge of results, this should – transferability being presupposed – be just as effective with imagined movements as with overt movements whose actual results, however, are not known by the subjects. Such a finding has been reported by Mendoza and Wichman [1978]. One group that practiced dart-throwing mentally made the same progress in performance as the second group who *did* perform the movements without actually throwing the darts (fig. 2).

A second problem dealt with in the literature is the effectiveness of imaginations of the results of imagined throwing movements, which may be regarded as a phenomenal correlate of an internal knowledge of results. Powell [1973] instructed his subjects to imagine precise throwing movements during periods of mental practice which alternated with periods of physical practice. In addition, one of the two experimental groups was to imagine the dart hitting the center of the board, whereas a second group was to imagine the dart hitting the edge. In the first group an improvement of 28 % was found, in the second group, however, a deterioration of 3 % – in spite of an improvement which was to be expected solely on account of the physical

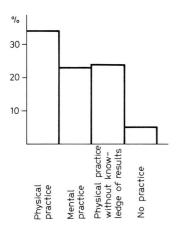

Fig. 2. Mental practice compared to physical practice without knowledge of results [from Mendoza and Wichman, 1978].

practice. Therefore, imaginations of the results modify the imagined throwing movements just as imaginations of the results of movements actually performed change these [Finke, 1979].

Conclusions

To summarize, there appears to be a major basis and a secondary basis for the beneficial effects of mental practice on the performance of motor skills. The major basis is the cognitive manipulation of symbolic and visuospatial representations that can be communicated without ever having performed the movement. The extent to which such cognitive manipulations are expressed in performance depends on the degree to which the representations can be transformed into motor commands. If transformation rules are known prior to mental practice, mental practice will be effective even if there has not been any preceding physical practice. Under these conditions 'motor learning' becomes purely 'cognitive learning' of symbolic and visuospatial representations which can directly be transformed into corresponding motor commands on the basis of the transformation rules already known. Mental practice may be even more effective than physical practice if the performance of movements distracts from 'cognitive learning' or interferes with the latter in any other way.

Mental practice is not likely to produce major benefits if the rules for transforming symbolic or visuospatial representations into motor commands are unknown. Learning such rules seems to require the experience of the correlations among the variables related by them [Heuer, 1983, chapt. 2, 3]. These correlations, however, can be experienced with tasks quite different from the one to be learned. Thus certain pretraining procedures can serve to establish those rules useful for subsequent mental practice.

The potential secondary basis of mental practice effects is repeated programming which accompanies imaginations of a motor pattern. An important but unsolved issue is whether this actually occurs and if so, under what conditions. It appears likely that programming is associated with kinesthetic imagery but not with visual imagery. Furthermore, correct kinesthetic imagery may not be possible for movement patterns for which appropriate motor commands are not available and which have never been performed. These, however, are speculations that have scarce experimental foundation; but they point to questions that need to be answered.

What are the practical implications of the multiple representations' approach to mental practice outlined in this chapter? The most obvious implication is that, although mental practice is frequently considered as an inferior substitute for physical practice, to be implemented in situations where the latter is impossible [e. g. Volkamer, 1972], it can be a superior mode of practice. This will be the case if acquiring a skill involves only learning symbolic or visuospatial representations and if actual execution of movement interferes with 'cognitive learning'.

A second implication is that mental practice will be of minimal or no use when rules are unavailable for transforming symbolic or visuospatial representations into motor commands. In this case, manipulations of these representations will remain isolated from the effector systems. Learning of transformations between representations seems in principle to require physical practice as there is no other way of learning whether an assumed correlation between two or more variables is actually correct. There is no way of knowing whether a certain set of motor commands will result in a certain seen or felt position of a limb except by executing them.

Simply stated, mental practice appears to be the better mode for learning symbolic or visuospatial representations, while physical practice appears to be necessary for learning how to transform these representations into motor commands. (Given a partially learned motor representation, mental practice appears also to operate on this to some degree.) Depending on what kind of learning is required, the relative benefits of both modes of practice will vary.

In many cases both kinds of learning are required. Then it may be useful to separate them by using mental practice trials, during which manipulations of symbolic or visuospatial representations can be performed without interference due to the demands of controlling movements, in combination with physical practice trials, in which transforming the modified representations into motor commands can be learned. The fact that combinations of mental and physical practice have been reported to be superior to physical practice alone suggests that the temporal separation of both kinds of learning can be beneficial.

A special learning situation arises after damage to the central nervous system due to traumata, cerebrovascular accidents, etc. Rehabilitation of these patients obviously represents a problem different from that posed by learning a new skill. Rather it is re-learning of old skills with partially changed characteristics of the central nervous system. There is some evidence that combining mental practice with more conventional rehabilitation procedures is beneficial for the patients [e.g. Guenther, 1980]. Several different mechanisms may underly these benefits, partly depending on the functional characteristics of the disturbance.

Firstly, mental practice may have nonspecific effects by way of enhancing motivation and effort. Although it may be impossible to perform a particular motor task physically, it might be motivating to be able to do it in an imaginary way. Second, mental practice after damage to the central nervous system may facilitate retention of remaining intact representations although they cannot be used for motor control until sufficient recovery has occurred. The potential function of maintaining existing representations implies activation of the corresponding neural substrates and might consequently further prevent physiological changes due to insufficient use. Finally, mental practice might improve the search for new strategies of moving a limb, in that the evaluation of a new strategy is postponed, just as the evaluation of an idea is postponed in 'brainstorming' procedures of problem-solving. In general, however, the basis of mental practice effects in the rehabilitation of central disorders of movement constitutes an as yet unsolved problem and a challenge to research.

References

Adams, J.A.: A closed-loop theory of motor learning. J. Motor Behav. *3:* 111–150 (1971).
Adams, J.A.: Do cognitive factors in motor performance become nonfunctional with practice? J. Motor Behav. *13:* 262–273 (1981).

Corbin, C.B.: Mental practice; in Morgan, *Ergonomic aids and muscular performance* (Academic Press, New York 1972).

Epstein, M.L.: The relationship of mental imagery and mental rehearsal to performance of a motor task. J. Sport Psychol. *2:* 211–220 (1980).

Feltz, D.L.; Landers, D.M.: The effects of mental practice on motor skill learning and performance: A meta-analysis. J. Sport Psychol. *5:* 25–57 (1983).

Finke, R.A.: The functional equivalence of mental images and errors of movement. Cogn. Psychol. *11:* 235–264 (1979).

Guenther, W.: Untersuchungen zur Wirksamkeit mentaler Trainingsverfahren grobmotorischer Bewegungen bei der Rehabilitation zentralmotorisch Behinderter. Diss. (Tübingen 1980).

Hein, A.; Held, R.: A neural model for labile sensorimotor coordinations; in Bernard, Kare, Biological prototypes and synthetic systems, vol. 1 (Plenum Press, New York 1962).

Heuer, H.: Bewegungslernen (Kohlhammer, Stuttgart 1983).

Heuer, H.: The laboratory and the world outside: in Meijer, Roth, Complex movement behavior: The motor-action controversy (North-Holland, Amsterdam 1988).

Heuer, H.; Prinz, W.: Initiierung und Steuerung von Handlungen und Bewegungen; in Amelang, Bericht über den 35. Kongress der Deutschen Gesellschaft für Psychologie, Heidelberg 1986 (Hogrefe, Göttingen 1987).

Heuer, H.; Wing, A.M.: Doing two things at once: Process limitations and interactions; in Smyth, Wing, Psychology of human movement (Academic Press, London 1984).

Jacobson, E.: Electrophysiology of mental activities. Am. J. Psychol. *44:* 677–694 (1932).

Kelso, J.A.S.: Motor control mechanisms underlying human movement reproduction. J. Exp. Psychol. *3:* 529–533 (1977).

Lashley, K.S.: The accuracy of movement in the absence of excitation from the moving organ. Am. J. Physiol. *43:* 169–194 (1917).

MacKay, D.G.: The problem of rehearsal or mental practice. J. Motor Behav. *13:* 274–285 (1981).

MacKay, D.G.: The problems of flexibility, fluency, and speed accuracy trade-off in skilled behavior. Psychol. Rev. *89:* 483–506 (1982).

McGuigan, F.J.: Covert functioning of the motor system; in Schwartz, Shapiro, Consciousness and self-regulation. Advances in Research and Theory, vol. 2 (Plenum Press, New York 1978).

Mendoza, D.; Wichman, H.: Inner darts: Effects of mental practice on performance of dart throwing. Percept. Mot. Skills *47:* 1195–1199 (1978).

Minas, S.C.: Mental practice of a complex perceptual motor skill. J. hum. Movem. Stud. *4:* 102–107 (1978).

Minas, S.C.: Acquisition of a motor skill following guided mental and physical practice. J. hum. Movem. Stud. *6:* 127–141 (1980).

Nissen, M.J.; Bullemer, P.: Attentional requirements of learning: Evidence from performance measures. Cogn. Psychol. *19:* 1–32 (1987).

Poulton, E.C.: On prediction in skilled movements. Psychol. Bull. *54:* 467–478 (1957).

Powell, G.E.: Negative and positive mental practice in motor skill acquisition. Percept. Mot. Skills *37:* 312 (1973).

Prinz, W.: Ideomotorik und Isomorphie; in Neumann, Perspektiven der Kognitionspsychologie (Springer, Berlin 1985).

Richardson, A.: Mental practice: A review and discussion. 1. Res. Q. *38:* 95–107 (1967a).

Richardson, A.: Mental practice: A review and discussion. 2. Res. Q. *38:* 263–273 (1967b).

Richter, H.: Über ideomotorische Phänomene. Z. Psychol. *157:* 201–257 (1954).

Richter, H.: Zum Problem der ideomotorischen Phänomene. Z. Psychol. *161:* 161–254 (1957).

Roland, P.E.; Larsen, B.; Lassen, N.A.; Skinhoj, E.: Supplementary motor area and other cortical areas in organization of voluntary movements in man. J. Neurophysiol. *43:* 118–136 (1980).

Ryan, E.D.; Simons, J.: Cognitive demand, imagery, and frequency of mental rehearsal as factors influencing acquisition of motor skills. J. Sport Psychol. *3:* 35–45 (1981).

Ryan, E.D.; Simons, J.: Efficacy of mental imagery in enhancing rehearsal of motor skills. J. Sport Psychol. *4:* 41–51 (1982).

Schmidt, R.A.: A schema theory of discrete motor skill learning. Psychol. Rev. *82:* 225–260 (1975).

Stimpel, E.: Der Wurf. Neue psychol. Stud. *8:* 105–138 (1933).

Taub, E.; Goldberg, I.A., Taub, P.: Deafferentation in monkeys: Pointing at a target without visual feedback. Expl. Neurol. *46:* 178–186 (1975).

Thomas, A.: Einführung in die Sportpsychologie (Hogrefe, Göttingen 1978).

Ulich, E.: Some experiments on the function of mental training in the acquisition of motor skills. Ergonomics *10:* 411–419 (1967).

Ungerer, D.: Zur Theorie des sensomotorischen Lernens (Hofmann, Schorndorf 1977).

Vandell, R.A.; Davis, R.A.; Clugston, H.A.: The function of mental practice in the acquisition of motor skills. J. gen. Psychol. *29:* 243–250 (1943).

Volkamer, M.: Bewegungsvorstellung und mentales Training; in Koch, Motorisches Lernen – Üben – Trainieren (Hofmann, Schorndorf 1972).

Wehner, T.; Vogt, S.; Stadler, M.: Task-specific EMG characteristics during mental training. Psychol. Res. *46:* 389–401 (1984).

Weimer, W.B.: A conceptual framework for cognitive psychology: Motor theories of the mind; in Shaw, Bransford, Perceiving, acting, and knowing. Toward an ecological psychology (Erlbaum, Hillsdale 1977).

Willimczik, K.; Poltz, M.; Fröhlich, H.; Rother, R.: Zur Effektivität des mentalen Trainings im Schulsport; in Letzelter, Müller, Sport und Sportwissenschaft (Bartels, Berlin 1976).

Wrisberg, C.A.; Ragsdale, M.R.: Cognitive demand and practice level: Factors in the mental rehearsal of motor skills. J. hum. Movem. Stud. *5:* 201–208 (1979).

Zecker, S.G.: Mental practice and knowledge of results in the learning of a perceptual-motor skill. J. Sport Psychol. *4:* 52–63 (1982).

Herbert Heuer, PhD, Fachbereich Psychologie der Philipps-Universität, Gutenbergstrasse 18, D–3550 Marburg (FRG)

Kirkcaldy B (ed): Normalities and Abnormalities in Human Movement.
Med Sport Sci. Basel, Karger, 1989, vol 29, pp 58–77

Childhood Sex Differences in Motor Performance and Activity Level: Findings and Implications[1]

Warren O. Eaton

Department of Psychology, University of Manitoba, Winnipeg, Canada

Childhood sex differences for many physical and motor measures are strikingly small in comparison to the same sex differences in adolescence and adulthood. As a consequence, it is widely assumed that prepubertal sex differences have a negligible role to play in various motor performance tasks. Is this assumption a reasonable and defensible one? Answers will be sought from recent quantitative reviews of empirical research with normal populations of children and adolescents.

A family of quantitative review procedures known collectively as 'meta-analysis' has emerged during the last 15 years and has aided greatly in the integration of research findings (for more information on meta-analytic procedures, see Halvorsen [1986], Light and Pillemer [1984], and Thomas and French [1986]). Because several of these quantitative reviews will comprise the core of this commentary, an overview of meta-analysis is in order.

Meta-Analysis

Essentially, meta-analysis is the statistical integration of the findings from many individual studies [Glass, 1977], and one of the major reasons for conducting such an integration is to determine the average size of a particu-

[1] The preparation of this chapter was supported by a grant from the Social Sciences and Humanities Research Council of Canada. The comments of J. Chipperfield, M. Eaton, N. McKeen, K. Saudino, and C. Singbeil on earlier drafts of this paper are gratefully acknowledged.

lar comparison [Light and Pillemer, 1984]. For present purposes, the comparison of interest is that between females and males, and the outcome of interest is the average size of the difference between them.

The Effect Size (ES)

The basic meta-analytic concept used in most sex difference reviews is the ES. For each female-male comparison a difference on the variable of interest can be calculated. However, because many different studies are typically included in a review, there are invariably different outcome measures. Thus, the magnitude of any difference must be translated from the various raw scales employed in the original research to some common metric for quantitative summary. The common metric is the ES, and the conversion is typically accomplished by dividing the difference between the means for males and females by a pooled standard deviation:

$$ES = (M_{male} - M_{female})/SD.$$

The ES is, in short, the sex difference comparison expressed in standard deviation units.

The average ES of all studies under review can be calculated to estimate a mean sex difference, or ES, for the variables or measures being integrated. Other analyses are also possible, e.g., various study characteristics can be related to ES. Typically, selected characteristics of the studies being reviewed are systematically coded and related to ES magnitude. For example, if the age of the subjects is thought relevant to the issue at hand, it could be correlated with ES. If sex differences enlarge with age, a positive correlation between age and ES would result.

The ability to estimate the strength of the relationship between a comparison and a variable of interest is an appealing advantage of meta-analysis over traditional review procedures. Rather than asking whether a difference exists, one asks how large the difference is. A difference of no magnitude (ES = 0.0) is, of course, one of the possibilities. Having estimated the size of a difference for a variable, one is inevitably drawn to compare its magnitude with those estimated for other variables. Such comparisons will be drawn here in the hope that they will inform our understanding of sex differences in motor behavior.

The expression of sex difference magnitudes in standard deviation units is, however, a mixed blessing because such an expression is very abstract and difficult to visualize. Fortunately, enough meta-analyses have been done so that it is now possible to place a particular sex difference into the context provided by gender differences for other variables.

The absolute magnitude of the ES indicates the size of a sex difference, and the algebraic sign of the ES indicates which group has the higher mean. Most reviewers have subtracted the female mean from the male mean for the variable in question. Hence, a positive ES reflects a higher male than female mean for the measure under review, whereas a negative ES reflects a higher female mean. This arbitrary convention will be continued to avoid confusion.

Statistical Significance

Statistical significance has often been confused with the magnitude or the importance of an effect [Ware et al., 1986]. A nonzero ES does not necessarily represent a statistically significant group difference. By the same token, a highly significant mean difference may represent a small ES. Given an ES of specified magnitude, the level of statistical significance will depend upon the sample size used. Ware et al. [1986] cite, as an example, the influence of a drug on cardiac index. If a treatment group, which received the drug, had a mean cardiac index that was 0.3 standard deviations (SD) higher than the mean for the untreated control group ($ES = 0.3$), the comparison would be statistically significant ($p < 0.05$) for a sample size of 100, but would be nonsignificant for a sample of 25.

It becomes apparent that the power to detect a difference that is statistically significant depends both upon the sample size and the magnitude of the difference between groups. Sample sizes can be so small as to make it unlikely that even a clinically meaningful group difference will result in a statistically significant difference. Frieman et al. [1986] found, for example, that many 'negative' outcomes in randomized clinical trials may have resulted from samples that were too small rather than from ineffective treatments.

Although meta-analytic studies tend to redirect one's attention from probability levels to ES magnitudes, questions of statistical significance can still be addressed. For example, the probability of obtaining a mean ES of a particular magnitude given the null hypothesis can be assessed. When reviewed studies are consistent as to the direction of the effect, i.e., one group displays consistently higher means across a sample of studies, even small mean ES's are statistically significant. Consequently, the size of the sex difference will be of prime concern throughout this chapter.

With this synopsis of meta-analysis as background, consider then the meta-analytic evidence for sex differences on motor performance tasks.

Sex Differences on Motor Performance Tasks

Motor development tasks in childhood and adolescence have been studied frequently over the years, and an adequate base of studies for a meta-analysis exists. Thomas and French [1985] applied meta-analytic procedures to this base to estimate sex differences in motor performance, which they defined as the outcomes of movement. They excluded measures of cardiovascular fitness and analyzed 20 outcome measures including: basic abilities such as balance and fine eye-motor coordination; information-processing responses such as reaction time and anticipation timing; fitness measures such as arm strength, flexibility, and sit-ups; and fundamental skills such as catching, throwing, running, and jumping.

Overall Sex Differences

Because many motor performance tasks show age-related changes in the size of sex differences, Thomas and French [1985] explicitly considered age as a covariate of sex difference magnitude. Thus, they required studies that included a female-male comparison and adequate information on the ages of the subjects. Sixty-four such studies were found, and these studies yielded 702 ES's based on 31,444 children and adolescents who ranged in age from 3 to 20 years. The number of ES's available for each task ranged from 13 to 85.

For the 20 tasks, the mean sex difference ES's are ranked in table I from those tasks on which females scored higher to those tasks on which males scored high. Thomas and French [1985] found significant sex differences on motor performance tasks in childhood and adolescence, but ES magnitudes varied considerably from task to task.

Developmental Patterns

Age was unrelated to the size of the sex difference for 8 of the 20 tasks. For most of the remaining tasks, ES's increased with age. For some, such as balance and vertical jump, there were no differences before puberty. For others, such as the long jump, prepubertal sex differences ranged from 0.2 to 0.5 SD and grew steadily larger with increasing age. For six of the tasks (dash, grip strength, long jump, shuttle run, sit-ups, and vertical jump), ES's increased dramatically at puberty and culminated in ES's of between 1.5 and 2.0 SD units at age 17. Throwing tasks were notable exceptions to the preceding patterns because they showed large sex differences prior to puberty, e.g., 1.5 SD at age 3. In summary, Thomas and French [1985] found

Table I. ES's for various motor performance measures from Thomas and French [1985] (adapted with permission)

Variable	Mean ES[1]	Pattern of difference across age
Flexibility	− 0.3	unrelated to age
Fine eye-motor coordination	− 0.2	unrelated to age
Arm hang	0.0	unrelated to age
Pursuit rotor tracking	0.1	no difference before puberty
Balance	0.1	no difference before puberty
Tapping	0.1	no difference before puberty
Vertical jump	0.2	no difference before puberty
Agility	0.2	unrelated to age
Reaction time	0.2	unrelated to age
Shuttle run	0.3	initially small, increases
Catching	0.4	declines, then increases
Anticipation timing	0.4	unrelated to age
Long jump	0.5	initially small, increases
Sit-ups	0.6	initially small, increases
Dash	0.6	initially small, increases
Grip strength	0.7	initially small, increases
Wall volley	0.8	unrelated to age
Throw for accuracy	1.0	unrelated to age
Throw for distance	2.0	initially large, increases
Throwing velocity	2.2	initially large, increases

[1] For ES's less than zero, females score higher; for ES's greater than zero, males score higher.

that sex difference magnitudes varied considerably from task to task, both in terms of overall level and in terms of developmental patterning.

In view of their exclusion from the Thomas and French [1985] analysis, cardiorespiratory sex differences need consideration. Unfortunately, such an analysis for children is not known to this author. However, Sparling [1980] has estimated adult sex differences for a basic cardiorespiratory measure, oxygen uptake, and has found male oxygen uptake capacity to exceed female capacity by 2.7 SD. Such a difference is very large in the context of differences reviewed thus far.

In discussing this large difference for oxygen uptake, Sparling [1980] noted that gender-associated differences in habitual motor activity level may play an important role in cardiorespiratory capacity. If present, sex differences in customary activity could also influence task performance variables by providing boys and girls with differential training. The question of sex differences in motor activity level has been addressed in a meta-analysis conducted by myself and Lesley Enns [Eaton and Enns, 1986], and it is to that analysis that we now turn.

Sex Differences in Motor Activity Level

Our interest in motor activity level was prompted by the role it plays in most theories of childhood temperament, not by its relevance for cardiorespiratory capacity or physical performance. Most theories of infant and childhood temperament [Buss and Plomin, 1984; Thomas and Chess, 1977] assign a prominent role to individual differences in activity level, and the question of sex differences in activity level had been raised but not resolved [Maccoby and Jacklin, 1974].

We viewed activity level from a trait perspective and defined it as the individual's customary level of energy expenditure through movement. Energy expenditure through movement can have many goals and be expressed in various ways. That variability notwithstanding, it is informative to consider individual differences in customary energy expenditure. As we viewed it, our definition of activity level is analogous to the concept of disposable income. Just as one's income can be spent for a variety of purposes and in a variety of ways, so too can one's energy be directed towards various goals and take on various forms. We do not hesitate in considering differences between the customarily rich and the customarily poor, and we can, in like manner, derive reasonable generalizations about differences in customary activity level.

A wide variety of motor activity measures have been used in research [Halverson and Post Gorden, 1984; Tryon, 1985], and diverse assessments were available for review. We included any activity measure that reflected energy expenditure through movement. Measures of movement frequency, duration, amplitude, and type could all affect the amount of energy expended, and all were utilized. Generally speaking, large, frequent, long-duration, and expansive movements require more energy than fine, infrequent, short-duration, and constricted ones. Specific limb movements as well as whole body actions were deemed acceptable.

While casting a wide net for studies of activity level, we restricted consideration to normal samples, and excluded subjects with reported pathologies, be they emotional, behavioral, physical, or mental. Consequently, samples of hyperactive children were not included. The control groups used in hyperactivity studies, however, often fulfilled our selection criteria and were included. In total, our review analysis was based on 90 publications, which comprised 127 independent comparisons of females and males on some measure of activity level.

Developmental considerations played a role in our review, just as they had in Thomas and French's [1985]. Maccoby and Jacklin [1974] had argued that sex differences in activity level were age-specific in that they were not to be found in infants under 1 year of age. If true, this would lead to the prediction of a positive correlation between the age of the sample and magnitude of the ES. Another line of reasoning led to the same prediction. If socialization processes, e.g., differential patterns of reinforcement for motor activity in males and females, are responsible for activity level sex differences, one would expect larger differences in older samples on the assumption that such learning processes take time to work. Differential socialization of the sexes would, we thought, lead to a positive relationship between age and ES. Although we did not restrict our analysis by age, most studies that were found were conducted with children. The mean chronological age of the study samples in the meta-analysis was 6.3 years.

Situational influences on activity level have been identified [Carpenter and Huston-Stein, 1980; Eaton and Keats, 1982], and one aspect of situational influence deemed important was the degree to which movement was controlled and restricted. We hypothesized that the size of a sex difference would be smaller in settings where movement was restrained. We consequently coded studies for the judged level of movement restriction in the measurement situation. We also coded the measurement setting for degree of stress and familiarity, two other situational variables thought to be important.

The level of objectivity with which activity level was measured was also coded for each sex difference comparison. We identified three categories of measurement techniques and ranked them from most to least objective as follows: instruments, observations, and ratings. If reported sex differences were subjective rather than real, ES magnitude was expected to vary with the degree of measurement objectivity; the largest and smallest ES's were hypothesized for ratings and instruments respectively.

Across all the studies the mean ES was 0.5 SD units, with males being more active. Such an outcome was highly unlikely to have occurred by chance, $z = 50.79$, $p < 0.0001$. Other statistical tests showed that the studies were not homogeneous, namely, it was unlikely that they all were manifestations of the same unobservable population ES. This prompted a search for characteristics of the studies that would correlate with ES magnitude.

One of the characteristics we thought would be important, measure objectivity, was not. Sex differences were no larger when based on observer ratings than when based on instruments, a finding that suggested to us that sex differences are not solely in the mind of the beholder. Several situational factors were significant correlates of ES. Generally, large sex differences were found when behavior was assessed in familiar, nonstressful, unrestrictive surroundings when peers were present. Age was positively correlated with ES, $r = 0.26$, $p < 0.01$, which meant that the magnitude of differences increased with age as hypothesized.

Activity level sex differences may well have implications for gender comparisons on motor performance tasks, because physical activity is important in the regulation of body composition and weight and in the integrity and growth of muscle and skeletal tissues [Malina, 1983]. For example, activity is strongly related to lean body mass [Thompson et al., 1982], which, in turn, plays a pivotal role in tasks requiring the movement of body weight [Sparling, 1980]. The presence of a sex difference in activity level in quite young children may, consequently, contribute to task performance differences that are present later when children are first assessed at 4 or 5 years of age.

The preceding suggestion prompts consideration of possible causes for sex differences. It must be emphasized that the meta-analytic results are descriptions, not explanations, of sex differences. Explanations should, of course, be consistent with the descriptive data, and it is to explanations that we now turn.

Explanations for Gender Differences

Keogh and Sugden [1985, p. 168] attribute gender differences in motor performance tasks to sex differences in biological makeup and in participation experiences. Disentangling these alternatives is particularly difficult in the absence of experimental control over each putative cause. Nevertheless, several approaches to the unraveling of biological and experiential causes have been attempted and will be described.

The Covariance Strategy

One strategy is to covary known biological sex differences from observed behavioral differences. Any difference remaining after such adjustment is presumably not due to the biological covariates. On the other hand, the reduction in the size of the difference is attributable to the covariates. For example, Sparling [1980] used a covariance strategy in his study of oxygen uptake. Mean male uptake was 2.7 SD greater than that of females. Physical size accounted for a large part of the observed difference, which decreased to 1.9 SD after adjustments for sex differences in body weight. When a body composition measure, relative fatness, was covaried, the ES shrank further to 0.6 SD. Thus, much – but not all – of the difference in oxygen uptake could be attributed to gender differences in body size and relative fatness.

Clark and Phillips [1987] used a related strategy by considering performance differences after making adjustments for physical size differences. They considered throwing, running, and balancing in 6-year-olds. For throwing performance, they substituted male forearm length and shoulder height values for female values in a prediction equation and found that the resulting predicted distance was short of the observed value for males. They also substituted male for female lower limb length values into a running speed equation and found the resulting predicted value to be less than the observed male running speed. Similarly, they substituted male for female values for center of gravity, foot breadth, and foot length in predicting performance on a static balance task. Once again the substitution did not bring a match between predicted and observed performance. They concluded, 'that anthropometric influences account for little of the gender-related performance differences in throwing, running and balance' [p. 176], and argued that alternative explanations must be sought.

Limb lengths are not the only possible biological variables that one could consider. Indeed, a key to the covariance strategy is the consideration of all the appropriate variables. The choice of the appropriate covariates can be difficult because the list of candidates is almost infinitely long. As a first step in such a choice, one should consider those covariates that display relatively large sex differences. For this reason, sex difference ES information for a variety of variables becomes quite useful.

It was possible to calculate performance, body size, and body composition ES's from a recent report by Nelson et al. [1986] on three aspects of throwing performance in 5-year-olds. Nelson et al. [1986] evaluated a number of physical variables, such as height and weight, and experiential variables, such as time spent playing with other children. ES's have been calculated for the data of Nelson et al. [1986] and are presented in table II.

The gender differences for three aspects of throwing performance were all quite large, and consistent with Thomas and French's [1985] meta-analytic results. Several indices of body composition and size also show large sex

Table II. Sex difference ES's for throwing performance, body size, and body composition variables in a sample of 5-year-olds

Variable	ES[1]
Throwing performance variables	
Distance	1.8
Trunk rotation	1.2
Foot action	0.9
Size and body composition measures	
Joint diameters	0.9
Sum of skinfolds	− 0.7
Endomorphy	− 0.6
Arm muscle	0.5
Forearm length	0.3
Height	0.2
Weight	0.2
Leg muscle	0.2
Shoulder/hip ratio	0.2
Arm length	0.1
Body mass index	0.0

[1] Calculated from published data in Nelson et al. [1986, tables 1–3]. Adapted by permission.

differences, which suggests their use as possible covariates in predicting throwing performance. Taken singly, however, most of the size and body composition differences are not as large as the throwing performance differences. It must be remembered, though, that several physical differences could operate additively or synergistically.

A wealth of potential ES information is currently available in compilations of published data [Malina and Roche, 1983; Roche and Malina, 1983]. For example, as a check on the representativeness of the Nelson et al. [1986] data, a sex difference ES was calculated for estimated upper arm circumference in US children from the Health Examination Survey [Malina and Roche, 1983, table 238]. The ES for 6-year-olds in that sample (the youngest age available) was 0.4 SD and reasonably close to the 0.5 value in table II for the same variable. Similarly, Nelson et al.'s [1986] sum of skinfolds measure produced an ES of − 0.7. The ES of 5-year-old subscapular skinfold thickness, one component of the sum of skinfolds variable, estimated from Malina and Roche [1983, table 322] was − 0.5. Existing information can provide a relatively untapped source of heuristic ES information for use with the covariate strategy.

Social factors could also relate to sex difference magnitudes. Nelson et al. [1986] reported that boys played more with other children than did girls, which suggested differential experience as a possible basis for throwing performance differences. ES information can be as useful for the consideration of experiential factors as for physical factors.

The Developmental Context Strategy

A second strategy for disentangling social and biological influences is to embed sex differences in a developmental context. The age at which sex differences appear or change dramatically is important because it has implications for the respective roles of biology and culture.

In considering the etiology of sex differences in activity level, we [Eaton and Enns, 1986] were interested in whether sex differences were present in the first year of life. They were. A difference at such a young age does not exclude experiential causes for a difference, but makes such an explanation less persuasive because learning usually takes time. Thus, the earlier the difference appears, the less time for learning, and the less plausible the role of social experience. The retreat into infancy is, however, much like a mirage. As you approach, the phenomenon recedes. Parents may respond differentially to male and female infants at quite a young age [Lewis, 1972; Moss, 1967], and in so doing provide a plausible experiential basis for sex differences in the first year of life. Thus, the contributions of biology and social factors are both present from the first days of postnatal life. In the case of activity level, we [Eaton and McKeen, 1987] are pursuing the issue into the fetal period to see if sex differences in activity level precede exposure to the social world.

Fetal studies are impractical for motor performance tasks, and the developmental strategy has focused on the developmental transitions of pubescence. For example, Thomas and French [1985] reasoned that synchronicity in the increase for a behavioral ES and the increase in sexual dimorphism implied a biological contribution to the behavioral sex difference. ES's for grip strength and long jump tasks widen abruptly in early adolescence, and as a consequence, biological contributions are strongly suspected. However, it is important to remember that even when performance and physical differences co-occur, social factors may overlay biological factors in contributing to the magnitude of sex differences [Thomas and French, 1985].

An interesting feature of Thomas and French's [1985] analysis is the argument that small prepubertal differences are probably environmental in origin. As Thomas and French [1985] put it: 'The differences prior to

Table III. Sex difference ES's from meta-analyses of selected behavioral and cognitive variables

Variable	ES[1]	Source
Empathy, self-report	− 1.0	Eisenberg and Lennon, 1983
Decoding nonverbal cues	− 0.3	Hall, 1978
Verbal ability	− 0.2	Hyde, 1981
Empathy, picture-story	− 0.1	Eisenberg and Lennon, 1983
Self-attributed responsibility	− 0.1	Cooper et al., 1981
Combinations	0.0	Meehan, 1984
Propositional logic	0.0	Meehan, 1984
Spatial visualization	0.1	Linn and Petersen, 1985
Proportional reasoning	0.3	Meehan, 1984
Spatial perception	0.4	Linn and Petersen, 1985
SAT mathematics performance	0.4	Rossi, 1983
Activity level	0.5	Eaton and Enns, 1986
Field articulation	0.5	Hyde, 1981
Aggressiveness	0.5	Hyde, 1984
Mental rotation	0.7	Linn and Petersen, 1985

[1] For ES's less than zero, females score higher; for ES's greater than zero, males score higher.

puberty are more moderate and, we believe, more likely to reflect environmental influences. When differences between the mean performances of boys and girls are less than 0.50 standard deviation units, many girls are performing better than many of the boys. If equal expectations, encouragement, and practice opportunities were provided by parents, teachers, and coaches, differences of this size could probably be eliminated' [p. 274].

The contention that '... physical characteristics of boys and girls are very similar prior to puberty' [p. 260] is central here. Certainly if this is true, it follows that '... biology seems to offer little explanation for motor performance differences prior to puberty' [p. 260]. But is it the case that prepubertal physical sex differences are too small to make a difference on motor performance tasks?

It is obvious that prepubertal sex differences in body size and composition are small relative to postpubertal differences. But are childhood physical differences small relative to other sex differences in the literature? Consider the context provided by other behavioral and cognitive differences that have been studied using meta-analyses. Table III presents a summary of such ES's. This list is by no means exhaustive, and glosses over many complexities in the comparisons of ES's, e. g., missing data may be treated differently from one analysis to the next. The summary is informative, nevertheless, because it illustrates the largely unappreciated fact that most well-established behavior-

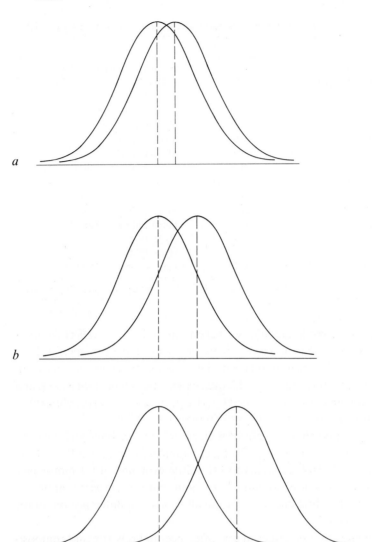

Fig. 1. Distribution overlap when ES = 0.5 *(a)*, ES = 1.0 *(b)* or ES = 2.0 *(c)*.

al and cognitive sex differences are substantially smaller than 1 SD in size. The ES for 5-year-old arm muscle in table II would not seem notably out of place in table III.

Recognition that prepubertal sex differences are comparable in size to other cognitive and behavioral sex differences means only that such differences are typical, not necessarily important. How, then, are we to interpret ES's of 0.5 SD? It is to that question that we now turn.

Interpreting Effect Sizes

The meaning of an ES is initially unclear, primarily because an abstract difference expressed in dimensionless standard deviation units is unfamiliar. Translation of ES's into more familiar terminology is a first, helpful step in interpretation, and several different translations are illustrated next.

Distribution Overlap

Consider figure 1a and the degree of overlap in the normal distributions of two groups when the means for the groups differ by 0.5 SD. The visual impression is clearly one of substantial overlap in the two distributions. We can translate that overlap into percentages [Cohen, 1969, p. 20], and upon so doing find that the upper 50% of individuals in one group exceed 69% of the individuals in the other group. If we were considering sex differences in activity, we would expect the average (median) boy to be more active than two-thirds of the girls. It would be simultaneously true that many girls would be more motorically active than the average boy.

Inspection of the distributions in the cases of larger ES produces a similar impression of substantial group overlap. Figures 1b and c depict the degree of overlap for ES's of 1.0 and 2.0 SD respectively. ES's of this magnitude are, however, salient without extensive research. Even young children notice that adult males tend to be taller than adult females, an ES of 1.8 SD (based on data for Canadian 18-year-olds, Roche and Malina [1983], table 71).

Correlation and Percentage of Variance

A second possible translation of an ES is into correlational terms. So considered, an ES of 0.5 becomes a correlation of 0.24. Squaring the correlation provides the percentage of total variance shared by the two variables. Thus, gender classification accounts for less than 6% of the total variance in activity. Six percent of the total variance does not sound like much to explain, and it is tempting to dismiss differences of this magnitude as unimportant [Hyde, 1981; Plomin and Foch, 1981].

Several considerations suggest that such a conclusion is premature. First, many widely accepted findings in the scientific literature are of this magnitude. Second, small amounts of explained variance enhance prediction to a surprising extent. Third, modest mean differences between two groups can produce dramatic differences in sex ratios at the extremes for the variable in question.

Living in Glass Houses

The reader who is ready to heave a stone at those trivial ES's smaller than 1 SD is advised to pause long enough to calculate the ES for a favored comparison. It is surprising to learn that many well-accepted and replicated findings in the scientific literature are not as large in magnitude as one would expect given highly significant probability levels [Hyde, 1981]. Consider some examples.

Examples of Effect Size Magnitude

One of the most famous series of studies in psychology was conducted by Milgram [1974], who asked research participants to administer what they believed to be damaging electric shocks to another participant. The level of subject obedience to the experimenter's instructions to continue to harm an innocent person has become one of the key findings covered in virtually all psychology textbooks. Funder and Ozer [1983] have re-expressed some of Milgram's effects into correlational terms, which in turn can be translated into the effect sizes as noted above. Two experimental manipulations that Milgram found to be important in influencing obedience were: (a) the extent of the subject's isolation from the victim, and (b) the proximity of the commanding authority. Based on Funder and Ozer's [1983] data, the ES's for the isolation and proximity manipulations were 0.9 and 0.8 respectively.

Perhaps ES's like Milgram's are more likely in 'soft' disciplines like psychology than in the 'hard' sciences [Hedges, 1987]. Are 'hard' empirical relationships of less than a standard deviation to be found? Certainly. The association between maternal smoking and infant birthweight is both firm and informative. This relationship is widely known and has been replicated in more than 45 studies [US Department of Health, Education and Welfare,

1979]. An ES calculated from the statistics of MacMahon et al. [1966], which were based on a sample of 12,193, indicates that the babies of nonsmoking mothers were heavier than the newborns of smoking mothers by 0.5 SD. If we were to discard as negligible all ES's of less than a standard deviation, the smoking-birthweight relationship would have to go.

Predictions at the Median

Prediction based on group membership of whether an individual would be above or below the median on an outcome variable is greater than one would suspect having looked at the degree of overlap in distributions. Rosenthal and Rubin [1982] have developed an intuitive, general technique for presenting ES's, the binomial effect size display. For a continuous outcome variable like activity level, one does a median split on the distribution of scores and then cross-classifies it with the category of interest, e.g., gender. Applying Rosenthal and Rubin's [1982] procedure to Thomas and French's [1985] sex difference ES of 0.5 for long jump performance, one would expect to find 38% of girls vs. 62% of boys to be above the overall median on long jump performance. Viewed from this perspective, 'small' effects begin to deserve respect.

Predictions at the Extremes

Small effects look larger yet if we shift our focus from the middle to the extremes of a distribution. Small differences in the means for two groups will translate into large differences in group representation at the extremes of the distribution. This phenomenon is exemplified by findings from several domains.

Mathematics Performance. Benbow and Stanley [1980] provoked a controversy when they reported large male-to-female ratios above extreme cut-offs on the mathematical portion of the Scholastic Aptitude Test, e.g., 5 males: 1 female above a score of 600. In criticizing Benbow and Stanley for exaggerating sex differences, Rossi [1983] calculated the ES for the Benbow and Stanley data and found it to be 0.44. The important point for our purpose is that a large ratio in group representation at the extremes can be consistent with mean differences that seem small when viewed in overlap or correlational terms.

Hyperactivity. Although there is disagreement about hyperactivity as a diagnostic entity [Achenbach, 1982; Knopf, 1984], the most common strategy for defining a group of 'hyperactive' children involves the use of an extreme cutoff score on an assessment instrument [Hinshaw, 1987]. For example, Schachar et al. [1981] had teachers and parents rate child activity on a 7-point scale. With a scale cutoff that identified 9% of the sample as hyperactive, the male-to-female ratio of those so identified was 2:1. This ratio was generated by an ES of 0.25. In clinical samples, which presumably represent more extreme selection criteria, the ratio of male-to-female hyper-actives ranges from 3:1 to 10:1 [American Psychiatric Association, 1980]. If Pascal [1966/1662] was right when he wrote that '... all men's misfortunes spring from the single cause that they are unable to stay quietly in one room', males would seem destined for more misfortune than females. In any case, it is once again evident that small mean group differences on a variable can translate into salient differences in group representation at the extremes for that variable.

Implications and Conclusions

Childhood sex differences in body size, body composition, and activity level are, with few exceptions, less than a standard deviation in size. However, not only are such ES's similar in magnitude to those found in other domains, they are too large to be dismissed as negligible in their potential influence.

The role for seemingly small ES's may well be greatest when extremes in performance are considered, as they inevitably are in competitive sports. In the context of athletic competition, differential representation of males and females will likely be largest where most attention is focused – on the outliers. It is relatively easy to notice whether a boy or a girl in a classroom is the most active, the most flexible, or the strongest. It is much more difficult to perceive the corresponding differences between the average girl and average boy on activity, flexibility, or strength. When children select peers for a game, they will remember whom is chosen first or last, not whom was chosen in the middle.

Beliefs about sex differences may well evolve from perceptions of extremes rather than from perceptions of average performance. Humans, young and old, are sensitive to the frequency of occurrence of events [Hasher and Zacks, 1984]. Exceptional levels of motor activity or performance are easily observed, and the frequency with which females and males are represented at exceptional levels may be a good candidate for such automatic encoding.

It must be emphasized that the differences described in this review are descriptive and do not, in and of themselves, imply biological determinism. If social influences are largely responsible for childhood sex differences on motor performance tasks, social changes may well lead to their reduction or elimination. Nevertheless, childhood sex differences in body size, body composition, and activity level are large enough to matter for motor performance tasks. Sex differences of less than a standard deviation are common in childhood and potentially more influential than they might first seem.

References

Achenbach, T.M.: Developmental psychopathology (Wiley, New York 1982).

American Psychiatric Association (APA): Diagnostic and statistical manual of mental disorders; 3rd ed. (APA, Washington 1980).

Benbow, C.P.; Stanley, J.C.: Sex differences in mathematical ability: Fact or artifact. Science 210: 1262–1264 (1980).

Buss, A.H.; Plomin, R.: Temperament: Early developing personality traits (Erlbaum, Hillsdale 1984).

Carpenter, C.J.; Huston-Stein, A.: Activity structure and sex-typed behavior in preschool children. Child Dev. 51: 862–872 (1980).

Clark, J.E.; Phillips, S.J.: An examination of the contributions of selected anthropometric factors to gender differences in motor skill development; in Clark, Humphrey, Advances in motor development research, vol. 1 (AMS Press, New York 1987).

Cohen, J.: Statistical power analysis for the behavioral sciences (Academic Press, New York 1969).

Cooper, H.M.; Burger, J.M.; Good, T.L.: Gender differences in the academic locus of control beliefs of young children. J. Pers. soc. Psychol. 40: 562–572 (1981).

Eaton, W.O.; Enns, L.R.: Sex differences in human motor activity level. Psychol. Bull. 100: 19–28 (1986).

Eaton, W.O.; Keats, J.G.: Peer presence, stress, and sex differences in the motor activity levels of preschoolers. Devl. Psychol. 17: 534–540 (1982).

Eaton, W.O.; McKeen, N.A.: Sex differences and longitudinal change in fetal activity level. Paper presented at the Society for Research in Child Development (Baltimore, April 1987).

Eisenberg, N.; Lennon, R.: Sex differences in empathy and related capacities. Psychol. Bull. 94: 100–131 (1983).

Frieman, J.A.; Chalmers, T.C.; Smith, H.; Kuebler, R.R.: The importance of beta, the type II error, and sample size in the design and interpretation of the randomized controlled sample; in Bailar, Mosteller, Medical uses of statistics, pp. 289–304 (New England Journal of Medicine Books, Waltham 1986).

Funder, J.C.; Ozer, D.J.: Behavior as a function of the situation. J. Pers. soc. Psychol. 44: 107–112 (1983).

Glass, G.L.: Integrating findings: The meta-analysis of research. Rev. Res. Educ. 5: 351–379 (1977).

Hall, J. A.: Gender effects in decoding nonverbal cues. Psychol. Bull. *85:* 845–857 (1978).

Halverson, C. F.; Post Gorden, J. C.: Measurement of open field activity in young children: a critical analysis; in Pollitt, Amante, Energy intake and activity, pp. 185–203 (Liss, New York 1984).

Halvorsen, K. T.: Combining results from independent investigations: Meta-analysis in medical research; in Bailar, Mosteller, Medical uses of statistics, pp. 392–416 (New England Journal of Medicine Books, Waltham 1986).

Hasher, L.; Zacks, R. T.: Automatic processing of fundamental information: The case of frequency of occurrence. Am. Psychol. *39:* 1372–1388 (1984).

Hedges, L. V.: How hard is hard science, how soft is soft science? The empirical cumulativeness of research. Am. Psychol. *42:* 443–455 (1987).

Hinshaw, S. P.: On the distinction between attentional deficits/hyperactivity and conduct problems/aggression in child psychopathology. Psychol. Bull. *101:* 443–463 (1987).

Hyde, J. S.: How large are cognitive gender differences? A meta-analysis using w^2 and d. *Am. Psychol. 36:* 892–902 (1981).

Hyde, J. S.: How large are gender differences in aggression? A developmental meta-analysis. Devl. Psychol. *20:* 722–736 (1984).

Keogh, J.; Sugden, D.: Movement skill development (Macmillan, New York 1985).

Knopf, I. J.: Childhood psychopathology; 2nd ed. (Prentice-Hall, Englewood Cliffs 1984).

Lewis, M.: State as an infant-environment interaction: An analysis of mother-infant interaction as a function of sex. Merrill-Palmer Q. *18:* 95–121 (1972).

Light, R. J.; Pillemer, D. B.: Summing up (Harvard University Press, Cambridge 1984).

Linn, M. C.; Petersen, A. C.: Emergence and characterization of sex differences in spatial ability: A meta-analysis. Child Dev. *56:* 1479–1498 (1985).

Maccoby, E. E.; Jacklin, C. N.: The psychology of sex differences (Stanford University Press, Stanford 1974).

MacMahon, B.; Alpert, M.; Salber, E. J.: Infant weight and parental smoking habits. Am. J. Epidem. *82:* 247–261 (1966).

Malina, R. M.: Human growth, maturation, and regular physical activity. Acta med. Auxol. *15:* 5–27 (1983).

Malina, R. M.; Roche, A. F.: Manual of physical status and performance in childhood, vol. 2 (Plenum, New York 1983).

Meehan, A. M.: A meta-analysis of sex differences in formal operational thought. Child Dev. *55:* 1110–1124 (1984).

Milgram, S.: Obedience to authority (Harper & Row, New York 1974).

Moss, H. A.: Sex, age, and state as determinants of mother-infant interactions. Merrill-Palmer Q. *13:* 19–36 (1967).

Nelson, J. K.; Thomas, J. R.; Nelson, K. R.; Abraham, P. C.: Gender differences in children's throwing performance: Biology and environment. Res. Q. Exercise Sport *57:* 280–287 (1980).

Pascal, B.: Pensées (A. J. Krailsheimer, Transl.; original work published 1662) (Penguin, Baltimore 1966).

Plomin, R.; Foch, T. T.: Sex differences and individual differences. Child Dev. *52:* 383–385 (1981).

Roche, A. F.; Malina, R. M.: Manual of physical status and performance in childhood, vol. 1 (Plenum, New York 1983).

Rosenthal, R.; Rubin, D.B.: A simple, general-purpose display of magnitude of experimental effect. J. educ. Psychol. *74:* 166–169 (1982).

Rossi, J.S.: Ratios exaggerate gender differences in mathematical ability. Am. Psychol. *38:* 348 (1983).

Schachar, R.; Rutter, M.; Smith, A.: The characteristics of situationally and pervasively hyperactive children: Implications for syndrome definition. J. Child Psychol. Psychiat. *22:* 375–392 (1981).

Sparling, P.B.: A meta-analysis of studies comparing maximal oxygen uptake in men and women. Res. Q. Exercise Sport *51:* 542–552 (1980).

Thomas, A.; Chess, S.: Temperament and development (Brunner/Mazel, New York 1977).

Thomas, J.R.; French, K.E.: Gender differences across age in motor performance: A meta-analysis. Psychol. Bull. *98:* 260–282 (1985).

Thomas, J.R.; French, K.E.: The use of meta-analysis in exercise and sport: A tutorial. Res. Q. Exercise Sport *57:* 196–204 (1986).

Thompson, J.K.; Jarvie, G.J.; Lahey, B.B.; Cureton, K.J.: Exercise and obesity: etiology, physiology, and intervention. Psychol. Bull. *91:* 55–79 (1982).

Tryon, W.W.: Measurement of human activity; in Tryon, Behavioral assessment in behavioral medicine, pp. 200–256 (Springer, New York 1985).

US Department of Health, Education and Welfare: Smoking and health: A report of the Surgeon General (US Government Printing Office, Washington 1979).

Ware, J.H.; Mosteller, F.; Ingelfinger, J.A.: P values; in Bailar, Mosteller, Medical uses of statistics, pp. 392–416 (New England Journal of Medicine Books, Waltham 1986).

Warren, O. Eaton, PhD, Department of Psychology, University of Manitoba, Winnipeg, Man. R3T 2N2 (Canada)

Kirkcaldy B (ed): Normalities and Abnormalities in Human Movement.
Med Sport Sci. Basel, Karger, 1989, vol 29, pp 78–99

Anxiety and Motor Performance

Peter Schwenkmezger, Georg Steffgen

Department of Psychology, University of Trier, FRG

Both common experience and scientific analyses show that attaining, maintaining and improving a certain performance level are not solely dependent upon talent and ability or, in the case of information reception and processing, upon cognitive processes. Learning and performance are accompanied by a number of motivational processes that arise as causes of behavior, consequences of behavior, or as accompaniments to behavior. This is true not only for performance in the cognitive area, but also for motor learning and performance. Because both motor performance and cognitive performance contribute to satisfying biological and socially-transmitted motives, failure to attain goals can be accompanied by emotions such as anxiety and anger. Movement-related fears can arise with motor actions that entail a certain risk of injury, but also with new and unknown tasks. Anxiety can also be expected to occur when failure to attain self-set or external goals is important to the person, i.e. when failure is relevant to self-esteem. This is particularly true when the social context seems to include other people's judgments or, in other words, when failure can be interpreted as making a fool of oneself in front of other people. Another issue that needs to be examined concerns the possibilities for anxiety control offered by motor performance.

Definitions

Anxiety can be regarded as a broad concept for a number of very complex emotional and motivational states and processes that occur as a result of a threat. This threat is related to the subjective evaluation of a situation, and concerns jeopardy to one's self-esteem during performance or social situations, physical danger, or insecurity and uncertainty.

If the anxiety reaction directly follows certain specific situational conditions, then anxiety is analyzed as a *state*. In this event three different levels of measurement have to be distinguished, as is usual in emotion research: the self-descriptive level, the physiological level and the behavioral level (further classified into avoidance and expressive behavior; cf. Hackfort and Schwenkmezger [1988]). One must also take into account the fact that the occurrence of state anxiety is tied up with experiential and behavioral processes, and can also be affected by the anticipation of imagined or real consequences.

Frequency of occurrence, probability of occurrence and intensity of the anxiety state are also dependent upon a chronic anxiety component, i.e. a *person-specific anxiety tendency* (trait anxiety). This tendency, which may also be influenced by phylogenetic developmental conditions, should be seen in relation to learning processes of habits or behavior dispositions in dealing with tasks, situations or environmental conditions [cf. Fröhlich, 1983, for an extensive discussion]. Other definitions focus on biological causes of anxiety reactions, and inherited differences in the reactivity of neural structures are held to be responsible for the existence of interindividual differences [Eysenck, 1981; Gray, 1982].

The second term in the title of this chapter, movement or motor behavior (the two words are used as synonyms here), comprises learning factors and performance-related processes that go along with the execution of a movement. Various different taxonomies of motor behavior are described in the literature. Fine motor behaviors are distinguished from gross motor behaviors, and discrete from continuous movements. Other points raised in definitions include relationships to type of task and individual performance abilities [Merrill, 1972], or the question of whether it is the person performing the action or the task- and situation-specific demands that determine the course of the movement (self-paced versus externally-paced motor behavior; cf. Poulton, [1957]).

Further attempts to systematize the structure of motor behavior have been made in the field of psychomotor research [e.g. Fleishman and Hempel, 1954], and in movement-related research or the analysis of movement in sports [e.g. Meinel and Schnabel, 1976; Hollmann and Hettinger, 1979]. Movements can be operationally defined by dividing them into specific motor behavior components, also called motor traits. Accordingly, motor performance can be assessed on the basis of quantitative product characteristics (e.g. speed, precision) and process characteristics (e.g. coordination).

With regard to the *course* of movement, quantitative characteristics – i.e., characteristics of the kinematic and dynamic movement structure – can be distinguished from qualitative movement characteristics (e.g. the rhythm of the movement, the flow of the movement) [Ballreich, 1983]. Qualitative components of movement are regarded as basic coordinative qualities. Obviously, these are very difficult to measure. Peterson [1985] notes that at most only the quantitative characteristics of qualitative movements can be examined and assessed with quantifying methods. Some of the approaches in this area include kinematographic analyses with high-frequency cameras, three-dimensional recording techniques and the precise recording of place and positional changes [Bös and Mechling, 1983]. Measurement instruments have yet to be developed for qualitative movement analyses.

Anxiety and Motor Performance

The effect of anxiety on motor performance is discussed on the basis of the following theories: learning and drive-theoretical approaches [Hull/Spence], the inverted-U function, cognitive approaches such as interference theories of anxiety, Spielberger's theory of anxiety and Martens' sport-specific modification, and the distinction between worry and emotionality. The relationship between anxiety and qualitative movement characteristics will be discussed and the results of a meta-analysis of the relationship between anxiety and sport motor performance is presented.

The Drive Theory Approach

One of the most important theories for the experimental analysis of anxiety and performance in the field of motor performance was developed on the basis of Hull's [1952] behavioristic theory. Space does not permit a detailed discussion of the theory here, and the reader is referred to the original works by Taylor [1956], Spence [1958], Spence and Spence [1966], as well as the comprehensive review by Krohne [1980].

In brief, the theory states that the strength of a specific behavior (B) is a function of the effective drive state (D) and habit strength (H): $B = f(D \times H)$.

The drive state is regarded as a hypothetical construct and defined as the sum of all of the energetic components affecting an individual at the time of the behavior. D is connected multiplicatively with habit strength. A habit is a relatively automatic sequence of reactions, mainly motoric. The hypothetical construct 'habit strength' represents the intensity of the tendency for a specific reaction to follow a certain stimulus.

In the case of anxiety this general behavior theory has been supplemented by the assumption that the drive level is dependent upon an emotional reaction that is caused by an aversive stimulus. There are individual differences in the strength of this emotional reaction. For the question of how the intensity of the emotional reaction (in this case, anxiety) should be operationalized, two possibilities are available: (1) Individuals can be classified according to their anxiety level on questionnaires. This method of operationalization is called the *chronic hypothesis*, since it is assumed that situation-independent differences in individuals' anxiety levels are responsible for any performance differences. (2) The second possibility is the induction of different situation-specific anxiety levels by applying stress stimuli, also known as the *situational* or *reactive hypothesis*.

Independent of these hypotheses variants it follows from drive theory that, as a result of low response competition, persons with high drive level will perform better on easier tasks than persons with a lower drive level [Krohne, 1980; Glanzmann, 1985].

In a comprehensive review, Martens [1971, 1974] summarized the results of studies in the field of motorics based on drive-theory postulates. His review included only those studies in which the Manifest Anxiety Scale (MAS) [Taylor, 1953] had been used to operationalize the anxiety level. Motor tasks included visual-motor discrimination tasks, tracking, fine-motor sorting, labyrinth tasks, ring throwing, flexibility, balancing and coordination tasks. Most of the designs permit a twofold evaluation of performance: amount and error frequency.

According to Martens' conclusions, high-anxious persons do indeed perform better on simple tasks, whereas low-anxious persons have an advantage executing difficult tasks. However, this is only true when the amount of performance per unit of time is used as the dependent variable. If one takes error frequency into account, then only a few studies show results that conform to the hypotheses.

If one combines the chronic and situational hypotheses and focus on those studies that distinguish between anxiety levels as well as taking account of the intensity of the aversive stimulus as an additional independent variable, the number of contradictory findings increases.

Hackfort and Schwenkmezger [1985] summarized findings reported in studies of sport motorics. Results concerning the chronic hypothesis, which postulates a connection between chronic forms of anxiety and sport performance level, are questionable methodologically and too inconsistent to allow a clear interpretation. As far as testing of the situative hypothesis is concerned, there are no studies in the sport motorics' field that satisfy high methodological standards.

Although comprehensive review articles do not permit any unambiguous conclusions to be drawn, psychophysiological constitution research does provide critical arguments against the chronic hypothesis. Myrtek [1975, 1982], for example, investigated relationships between parameters of physical endurance and psychological factors such as emotional lability, physical complaints and manifest anxiety. Classification analyses revealed four different groups: group 1 describes itself as not very anxious, and displays low endurance ability in the physical area; group 2 also describes itself as being low in anxiety, but has a high physical endurance ability; group 3 displays high anxiety levels and high physical stress endurance, and group 4 is characterized by high anxiety levels, coupled with little physical performance ability. The fact that the sizes of the four groups identified in the independent groups were almost equal shows that there is no general relationship between physical performance level and anxiety or emotional lability in psychophysiological constitution research. This is confirmed by large correlational studies, partly covering the same data, reported by Fahrenberg et al. [1979].

With process-oriented approaches, the course of the learning process has to be considered as well as the absolute performance level. At the beginning of the learning process, high-anxious persons should perform less well, because for them the task is still difficult. In later stages this task becomes increasingly easier, so that learning progress and level may increase more sharply in anxious individuals. In general psychological tasks in which the learning tasks involve verbal material or problem-solving, the hypothesis was confirmed when, in addition to the differentiation according to anxiety level, psychological stress stimuli were used to increase situative anxiety [Krohne, 1980].

The complexity of the relationships involved is illustrated by one of our own studies [Schwenkmezger, 1980, 1981]. We were able to show that in learning a gross-motor task, skiing, state anxiety at the beginning of the learning process depends solely upon the trait-anxiety level, probably due to lack of specific experience. With increasing learning progress, however, task-specific cognitions concerning the difficulty of the task or situation-specific judgments of external circumstances of the learning task (steepness of the hill, snow properties, weather, etc.) determine the intensity of the state-anxiety level. At the same time, the influence of trait anxiety decreases. This demonstrates that the interaction between chronic anxiety level, situation-specific stress stimuli, task difficulty and situation-specific conditions of learning and performance is still, for the most part, largely unexplored, at least in the gross motor area. These findings also expose extremely difficult methodological problems, because they show that cross-sectional studies always portray only individual time segments, and the results are clear and generalizable only when the exact circumstances at the time of assessing anxiety and motor performance are known. This also holds true for the question of the point in the course of the learning process at which a study takes place. Unless the experimental subjects are carefully chosen, there will probably be great heterogeneity in the sample so that, as in our study, the relationships are probably obscured as a result.

The Inverted-U Function

When discussing the relationship between anxiety and motor perform-ance, an inverted U-shaped relationship is frequently postulated, as in the Yerkes-Dodson law. Yerkes and Dodson [1908], in fact, only studied the relationship between arousal and performance in animals. In drawing paral-lels between arousal and performance, and anxiety and performance, in addition to problems associated with generalizing from animal results to humans, at least one additional assumption is required – namely, that anxi-ety is an indicator of arousal. If one overlooks these difficulties, then, accord-ing to Fiske and Maddi [1961], there is good reason to assume that the optimal arousal level required for solving a task is dependent upon the task's complexity. The optimal arousal level is higher for simple tasks than for more complex ones. An arousal level that produces optimal performance with a simple task may lead to impairment in complex tasks.

On the basis of the Yerkes-Dodson law Martens [1975] was able to demonstrate that different physiological arousal levels are necessary for dif-ferent sport tasks, if the aim is optimal performance. The differentiation is made according to the proportion of gross- or fine-motor movements. Gross-motor movements require a high level of physiological arousal, where-as fine-motor movements require less.

Landers [1980] took up a suggestion made by Martens [1974] and at-tempted to explain the inverted-U relationship between anxiety and performance using Easterbrook's [1959] cue-utilization theory. Easterbrook postulates the following conditions: (1) Level of performance is proportional to the number of cues utilized. (2) The number of cues utilized is inversely proportional to the level of emotional arousal. Under the additional assumption that (a) the simultaneous use of task-relevant and task-irrelevant cues reduces effectiveness and (b) in perception, irrelevant stimuli are eliminated before relevant stimuli, several conclusions may be drawn. Persons under a low level of arousal have a broad perceptual range, motivational deficits (e. g. lack of effort), or a low selectivity of relevant cues. In this case, performance is low. Perceptual selectivity increases with increasing arousal. Irrelevant cues are eliminated and performance improves. Increases in arousal beyond this optimal level lead to a further perceptual narrowing with elimination of task-relevant cues, and performance decreases, in accordance with the inverted-U hypothesis.

A chronic and a situational hypothesis can also be formulated for studies on the inverted-U function. For this reason it is important to vary both the person-specific anxiety level *and* the situation-specific stress level. Such studies have been conducted by Martens and Landers [1970], Weinberg and Ragan [1978] and Sonstroem and Bernado [1982]. The results of these studies do not contradict the Yerkes-Dodson law. However, no alternative hypotheses were thoroughly tested in these studies.

Despite the plausibility of the inverted-U function, it must be noted that there are very few empirical results on its validity in the motor area. Statements depicting this nonlinear relationship as a well-confirmed scientific principle [e. g. Cratty, 1967] are certainly premature, and more experimental studies are urgently required.

Cognitive Theories

Cognitive psychological analyses of the relationship between anxiety and performance do not reflect a unitary group of theories. Distinct from the more mechanistic viewpoint underlying drive theory, cognitive theories emphasize, in addition to person-related variables, evaluation of the situation, demands of the given task, and the person's own resources [Krohne, 1980]. In the following discussion, several important cognitive theories on anxiety will be presented, followed by an analysis of their contribution toward tracing the association between anxiety and motor performance.

As early as Sarason's studies in 1960 and 1978 a cognitive interpretation was suggested for the relationship between anxiety and performance, in the form of the inference theory. Sarason proposed that a distinction should be made between task-irrelevant and task-related cognitions in performance situations. Whereas task-irrelevant cognitions (e.g. feelings of inadequacy, fear of failure, a desire to avoid the situation) impair performance, task-related cognitions serve rather to enhance the quality of performance. This can best be illustrated by an experiment carried out by Sarason [1978]. Based on their scores of test anxiety on a questionnaire, the participants were divided into groups of high- and low-anxious subjects. Subjects were then assigned to 1 of 5 groups, which differed according to the type of instruction received: (1) performance-oriented instruction (the subject was told that his own ability would be tested); (2) task-oriented instruction (the subject was told that it was the task itself that was being studied); (3) motivation-oriented instruction (the subject was told that the study concerned determining learning curves in psychological experiments); (4) anxiety-reducing instruction, and (5) neutral instruction (control group).

It was clearly shown that in situations with strong emphasis on performance, subjects high in test anxiety reacted with a significant decrease in performance. Less anxious subjects produced the best performance in this situation. In contrast, subjects with high test anxiety demonstrate a significant increase in performance in situations that are unrelated to performance. This is especially evident when the highly anxious subjects are calmed by instruction or when they are allowed to watch the solving of sample tasks beforehand. In general, it was shown that performance orientation on its own does not always lead to a decrease in performance; this is only true for subjects with high test anxiety. These results, which have been confirmed time and again in other studies by the Sarason group, also offer clues about the optimal design of a performance situation depending upon the person-specific anxiety level. Even though the instructions given in psychological experiments sometimes seem artificial and not directly generalizable to reality, these results are important confirmation of the need to take into account individually optimal conditions in performance-test situations. Indeed, the requirement of test fairness demands this.

It remains to be shown that these results can be generalized to the field of motorics, but there is some favorable evidence. Späte and Schwenkmezger [1983], for example, in comparing training games and selection games in handball, observed an anxiety x situation interaction with regard to performance: under selection conditions high-anxious persons are more likely to perform poorly, whereas situational conditions are largely performance-irrelevant for low anxious persons. The case of the person who is a world champion during training but fails in a competitive situation is supportive evidence for the generalizability of Sarason's results.

Spielberger's Anxiety Theory and
Its Sport-Specific Modification by Martens

Spielberger's [1966, 1972] state-trait anxiety model has been cited most often over the past 15 years. Although it has been modified and expanded in many details, its basic form still holds. Countless studies, including the motorics' domain, have selected this model as their theoretical basis. For this reason the discussion of this theory will be dealt with more extensively.

The central feature of the theory is the distinction between trait anxiety and state anxiety. This provides a theoretical framework for the inconsistent distinction between chronic and situational anxiety in drive theory.

State anxiety is defined as a temporary emotional condition of the human organism that varies in intensity and is unstable with regard to time. It is described as consisting of subjective, consciously perceived feelings of tension and anxious expectancy, combined with an increase in activity of the autonomic nervous system. The anxiety-state reaction increases in situations which the individual perceives as threatening, whereby the subjective evaluation of threat does not necessarily correspond to objective danger.

The concept of *trait anxiety* depicts relatively stable individual differences in susceptibility to anxiety reactions, i.e. in the tendency to perceive a broad spectrum of situations as dangerous or threatening. Trait anxiety also reflects individual differences in the frequency and intensity with which anxiety states have occurred in the past and provides information about the probability that they will occur in the future [cf. Nitsch, 1981, on the intensity or extensity of stress susceptibility].

An anxiety state is induced when, during the evaluation process, an external stimulus is recognized as being threatening. Evaluation is dependent upon trait anxiety, as well as upon inner organismic states and biological needs. Testing of reaction alternatives available to the individual for coping with the threat also plays a part in the evaluation process. Thus, defence and adaptation processes can reduce the level of state anxiety. When such alternatives are not available, the level of state anxiety has a direct effect on behavior.

High-anxious persons, in contrast to low-anxious persons, tend to respond to threatening situations with a *sharper increase* in state anxiety. However, how this abrupt increase works, exactly is still an unanswered question [cf. Schwenkmezger, 1985a, for a detailed discussion]. In addition, only a very limited range of validity has been demonstrated for the trait-state anxiety model, since it only concerns situations relevant to self-esteem. It provides no predictions for physically threatening situations [Spielberger, 1972].

Schwenkmezger [1985a] analyzed relevant findings in the literature on the validity of the model and presented evidence from his own empirical studies, primarily from the field of sport motorics. He was able to show that the interaction effect, conforming to the model, occurred under an experimentally-induced but rather weak or medium form of ego-threat but did not occur under massive threats to self-esteem, as manifested in natural settings (e.g. real examination situations). This was also true for motoric and sport-specific performance tests.

Threats to self-esteem occur because the individual knows the costs of failure (such as a damaged self-image, injured self-esteem, reduced social approval, material loss resulting from delay in finishing school, university, or professional training), either from previous experience or by watching or hearing from others. Because these consequences are anticipated, such a situation can be characterized as threatening in the sense of Lazarus and Launier's [1978] definition.

Under conditions of a relatively mild ego-threat, the individual has a wider range of interpretations to choose from. The situation is minimally structured, and the subjects often are not able to perceive a threat in a self-esteem relevant interpretation. In high-anxious persons such circumstances may lead to mediating processes such as insecurity and disquiet and allow them to respond with a sharper increase in state anxiety. Low-anxious persons regard the situation as less threatening, since in general no real consequences occur in laboratory experiments. If, on the other hand, one enters a situation of ego-threat without this wide range of possible interpretations (e.g. actual test situations), then ego-threat becomes evident and subjects react with an increase in state anxiety, independent of their trait anxiety level. The only difference is in the initial level of state anxiety, which is lower for low-anxious persons. The result is parallel increases. This hypothetical relationship is depicted in figure 1.

In comparing this version with Spielberger's original model, it is evident that only a partial revision has been made. In the low and medium areas of the threat continuum there are differential increases which are larger for high-anxious persons than for low-anxious persons. Only in the area of extreme self-esteem threat parallel increases can be observed. This revised model explains why, for relatively mild, experimentally-induced threats,

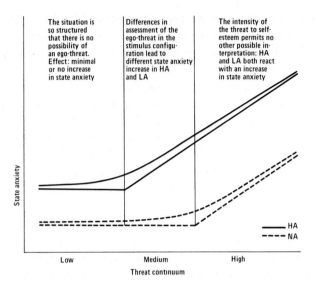

The situation is so structured that there is no possibility of an ego-threat. Effect: minimal or no increase in state anxiety

Differences in assessment of the ego-threat in the stimulus configuration lead to different state anxiety increase in HA and LA

The intensity of the threat to self-esteem permits no other possible interpretation: HA and LA both react with an increase in state anxiety

State anxiety

————— HA
- - - - NA

Low   Medium   High

Threat continuum

Fig. 1. Schematic course of the increase in state anxiety dependent upon trait anxiety. HA = High-anxious subjects; NA = low-anxious subjects. Modified from Schwenkmezger [1985a].

interaction effects occur in the sense of a steeper rise in state anxiety with high-anxious persons, whereas under strong actual threat situations more uniform increases are observed.

It is interesting that Eysenck et al. [1987], in a completely independent analysis, reached a conclusion similar to the proposed revision of the model. Their comparison of cognitive processes in high- and low-anxious individuals shows that high-anxious persons tend to approach threatening stimuli, whereas low-anxious persons tend to avoid such situations. These differences were found only under very specific conditions – for example, when threatening and nonthreatening stimuli were simultaneously present or when the threats were mild. According to the authors, there was no difference with massive threats.

Martens [1977] translated Spielberger's theory into the area of motorics, particularly to the situation of sport competition. Over the course of their sport-related learning history, individuals can develop a tendency to react with different amounts of anxiety in competitive sport situations. Martens postulates a sport-specific anxiety disposition; the Sport Competition Anxiety Test (SCAT) is an attempt to operationalize this disposition. People with a higher degree of this anxiety tendency are inclined – primarily in competitive situations – to perceive stimuli as threatening and, compared to people with a lower degree of anxiety, react with a significant increase in state anxiety. Consequences of this reaction include impairment of subjective well-being, physiological anxiety reactions and changes on the behavioral level (e.g. decreased performance). However, several analyses [Schwenkmezger, 1979] and studies by Singer and Ungerer-Röhrich [1985] have demonstrated that Marten's sport-specific anxiety test is no better at predicting state anxiety or motor performance than a more general measure of anxiety, for example the STAI by Spielberger et al. [1970]. Moreover, conformity to the model was not always demonstrated when this area-specific scale was implemented [cf. Hackfort and Schwenkmezger, 1988, for a summary of findings on this issue].

Distinguishing Emotionality and Worry

Liebert and Morris [1967] showed that state anxiety does not necessarily represent a homogeneous construct, but can be differentiated into two components, emotionality and worry. Worry is described as a cognitive process that takes place prior to, during, and following the execution of a task. Definitional elements include little faith in one's own performance, a high degree of worry, cognitions concerning the comparison of one's own performance with that of others, cognitions concerning the consequences of failure, and worrying about the effects of preparation on the self-esteem-relevant event. Emotionality, on the other hand, consists of affective-physiological symptoms caused by an increased arousal level (nervousness, faster heartbeat, stomach pains, feeling unwell, insecurity, and panic attacks).

Liebert and Morris [1967] treat emotionality and worry as co-components of state anxiety, whereas Wine [1971, 1980, 1982] hypothesizes that there is high intraindividual stability with regard to worry. It follows from this statement that she feels the worry component has the status of a more situation-specific trait. High-anxious persons, therefore, are inclined to worry about their poor performance and be distracted from the task they were involved in, with the result that the time available for them to solve the task is reduced. In substance, the worry reaction is largely identical to the definition proposed by Liebert and Morris [1967].

With regard to the theoretical foundations for distinguishing between the two components, Morris et al. [1981] have suggested several supplements for showing that both components can be defined at the trait level as well as situation-specifically. Thus, emotionality can be regarded as a *physiological* reaction that, when operationalization takes place in the self-descriptive medium, reflects verbal representation patterns of physical reactions. These are induced on the one hand by habitual components described as conditioned emotional reactions to test situations and vary individually depending upon the person-related learning history. Conversely, situation-specific stimuli like noxious stimuli, the presence or absence of other persons, etc. also contribute to producing physiological reactions.

The occurrence of the worry reaction, on the other hand, is explained as a complex *cognitive* process. Person-specific components include learned patterns of thinking about oneself, about one's own personal ability, and about anticipated result expectancies in potentially threatening situations. The concern with oneself, negative self-evaluation and negative performance expectations are learned by experiencing success and failure, by feedback of evaluations and in comparisons of one's own performance with that of other people. On the one hand this social learning history determines a habitual worry component, but there are also situational circumstances that evoke worry cognitions, that can be deduced from the current evaluation of the situation. One consequence of these considerations as regards measurement theory is the need to construct trait and state scales for both components.

In several studies of performance tests in school and college, Deffenbacher [1980] showed that there is a medium-sized correlation between measures of worry components and performance indices; usually negative correlations between -0.30 and -0.50 have been found. In these studies, performance parameters did not correlate with measures of emotionality. Similar results were reported by Hodapp et al. [1982]. Of particular interest in this connection are causal analyses, as published by Hodapp [1982]. These confirmed the performance-reducing role of the worry components and also provided indications of possible performance-enhancing effects of the emotionality components.

The fact that some anxiety questionnaires combine worry and emotionality items may be another reason for the nonuniform results reported so far. Future studies should carry out the operationalization of worry and emotionality separately. Hodapp's results also illuminate new ways of approaching this question. Worry may be conceived of as a variable representing cognitive evaluation processes that may be suitable for predicting the performance result. This probably has the form of a linear relationship. Emotionality, on the other hand, could be an indicator of arousal; closer analysis may also reveal curvilinear relationships, e.g. in the form of an inverted-U function.

What Role Does This Theory Play in the Motor Domain?

One of the first analyses of the importance of distinguishing between emotionality and worry in the field of motor abilities was presented by Morris et al. [1975]. Different performance levels of typing accuracy and typing speed were examined; it was found that, while indicators of emotionality had no relationship whatsoever to performance level, worry components produced negative relationships. This result was consistent, independent of performance level.

The usefulness of the differentiation between worry and emotionality in the analyses of sport-related fears was demonstrated in some of our own studies. In one contribution [Schwenkmezger, 1985a], comprehensive correlational results are presented. They reveal that worry cognitions about competence, fears of failure, norms, and comparisons of one's own performance with that of others, covary negatively with performance in a performance test in track and field sports, even on the individual item level. No such relationships were found for emotionality items. Using an activity-specific scale measure of task-unrelated cognitions in a study of handball players, Schwenkmezger and Laux [1986] found that high-anxious players tend to have more task-unrelated cognitions than low-anxious players. In evaluation situations (selection games with evaluation of individual performance) there was a significant increase in task-unrelated cognitions compared to training situations. These results support Spielberger's state-trait model of anxiety. In addition, highly significant correlations were found between frequency of task-unrelated cognitions and assessments of individual performance by independent raters.

These results confirm the hypotheses formulated by Mahoney and Avener [1977], Endler [1978] and Martens [1978].

Anxiety and Motor Performance: A Qualitative View

The relationship between anxiety and motor performance has been examined primarily from a purely quantitative viewpoint in the theories analyzed so far, where the effect of anxiety has been measured solely on the result of movement. The influence of anxiety on the course of movement has been largely neglected. To illustrate this research field, focussing on variables of the course of movement, we shall discuss the works of a research group centered around Weinberg [1977] and the results of Allmer's [1982, 1983] analyses.

In the studies by Weinberg [1977], and Weinberg and Hunt [1976], four electromyographic variables were used to assess movement quality: *anticipa-*

tion referred to the increase in amplitude from baseline to major muscle contraction as measured in seconds. *Perseveration* was indicated by continued contraction of decreasing amplitude to the baseline following major muscle action, as measured in seconds. The sequence of muscle action was a comparison of onset time of major muscle contraction, of agonist and antagonist: *co-contraction* referred to simultaneous contraction of the muscles and *sequential contractions* to the sequential action of each group of muscles in the movement [also see Hunt and Massey, 1977].

In an induced failure situation (failure feedback) these indicators revealed significant differences in the course patterns, so that a discriminant analysis separation of high- and low-anxious persons resulted in 95% correct classifications. It is therefore not surprising that performance results using a gross-motor task (throwing tennis balls at a target), also revealed differences between high- and low-anxious persons.

In a later study with a similar design, Weinberg [1978] investigated the effects of success feedback as well as failure feedback. Both 'performance result' and the 'pattern of neuromuscular coordination' served as dependent variables. For both groups of variables it was shown that high-anxious persons yield better performance results and more favorable coordination patterns under success feedback, whereas low-anxious persons exhibit better performance results under failure feedback. This significant trait anxiety × feedback interaction was confirmed in another study [Weinberg, 1979].

From an action theoretical background, Allmer [1982] was interested in the effect of anxiety on motor learning and execution of movement. His general hypothesis was that anxiety alters the psychological and physical bases of movement regulation and thus hinders optimal movement behavior. Allmer differentiated between behavior-related anxiety indicators related to the *movement task* and those related to the *movement activity*. Examples of anxiety indicators for the movement task are task avoidance, task modifications, and task simplifications. For movement activity, these are movement inhibition, movement interruption, unsatisfactory flow of movement or an overhasty execution.

In a pilot study, Allmer [1983] attempted to find empirical evidence for this hypothesis. Under anxiety-reducing and anxiety-inducing conditions, children had to perform a particular motor task on the trampoline. In the anxiety-reducing condition the trampoline was further covered by a mat to avoid the risk of injury; these measures were not taken in the anxiety-inducing condition. In this study, therefore, the aspect of *fear of injury* was clearly the main focus. Movement characteristics such as angle between thigh and body, and between arm and upper torso at the point of maximum height of the jump were selected as dependent variables. The results revealed that body and arm angles were significantly less favorable in anxiety-inducing situations than in anxiety-reducing situations.

Interpretation and methodological analysis of this type of approach is problematical. If one were interested in determining precisely the optimal body angle for a movement execution, then kinematographic analyses with high-frequency cameras would be more suitable allowing for precise measurement of positional changes [Bös and Mechling, 1983]. In addition, it seems possible that, with this particular anxiety-inducing condition which did in fact increase the risk of injury, the changed body angle more likely represents a (possibly reflexive) protection mechanism, and can scarcely be interpreted as an anxiety indicator. As for interpretation, one must also ask whether movement anomalies point unambiguously to anxiety as a cause, instead of simply reflecting differences in the learning process, performance level or even in the person's ability to cope with anxiety.

Studies like these have earned our thanks for deflecting the focus of the anxiety-performance relationship away from the somewhat one-sided performance result aspect, towards qualitative elements of movement into our way of thinking. The studies described here, however, further demonstrate some of the weaknesses of this type of investigative approach. Methodological difficulties in assessing coordinative parameters were mentioned earlier. The registration of electromyograms is subject to artifacts, especially with gross-muscle activity. Moreover, optimal coordination is generally a prerequisite for the quality of a movement result. But this can usually be quantified in a highly reliable and valid form. The question arises, therefore, whether it is necessary to make the detour involving qualitative parameters, which are certainly more dubious with respect to test theoretical criteria. These difficulties are particularly apparent in the studies by Weinberg and Hunt [1976] and Weinberg [1977]: the electromyographic variables are only used for a discriminant analysis to distinguish between high- and low-anxious persons, whereas for the theory-related conclusions preference is given to the quantitative performance of the target-throwing task.

Anxiety and Sport Performance: A Meta-Analysis

Independent of theoretical orientation or the question of whether to use indicators of the performance result or the quality of the movement, one is of course left with the problem of how to summarize all of the empirical results regarding the relationship between anxiety and motor performance. Review articles published so far [e.g. those by Martens, 1971, 1974; Landers, 1980, or Hackfort and Schwenkmezger, 1985], as well as summaries in individual articles [e.g., Hackfort, 1983; Bös and Mechling, 1985, or Schwenkmezger, 1985a] do not yet permit a definitive answer. As far as the review articles are concerned, this is at least partly due to inadequate methodology. For example, Martens' conclusions are based on a so-called 'vote-counting' technique: i.e., a tally is made of studies that support a theory and those that do not. This method can lead to statistically false conclusions [Schwarzer, 1987; Kleine, 1988]. The single studies suffer from the fact that they are frequently interpreted by their authors with respect to their theoretical statements, whilst the pragmatic question about what kind of relationship *does* exist between anxiety and motor performance tends to remain unanswered. Often the anxiety measures and the performance indices that have been implemented are much too heterogeneous to permit any comparative results whatsoever. Yet another problem lies in the sometimes very specifically constructed anxiety measures. For example, the correlation coefficients reported by Bös and Mechling [1985] must be viewed against the fact that extremely specific anxiety measures were used, and as a result there is a danger of *criterion confounding* – i.e., a close relationship is to be expected because of the similarity between predictor and criterion.

The only promising method remaining, then, is a meta-analysis. Like Schwarzer et al. [1987], who summarized results concerning mathematics' performance and anxiety, Kleine [1988] undertook a meta-analysis of the relationship between anxiety and sport performance. He analyzed results from a total of 37 studies, 58 independent samples and 3220 subjects, and subjected these results to a meta-analysis of the effect sizes. He differentiated according to sex, type of anxiety measure (sport-specific versus general), type of sport and time at which the anxiety measurement was taken.

The most important findings of Kleine's analysis can be summarized as follows: Not a single effect size was on the positive side: anxiety and sport performance covary consistently negatively. Effect sizes were significantly greater for male subjects than for females. Sport-specific tests did not explain a larger proportion of variance than general tests of anxiety. In addition, the worry-emotionality distinction was found to be important in this study: there were significantly greater effects for worry. The time at which anxiety was measured was also influential: longer intervals produce smaller effect sizes, but if anxiety is measured directly prior to the performance test, the relationships are closer. The largest effect sizes are observed when anxiety indicators are measured directly following the performance test. In this event, however, the causal relationship is probably reversed, since a failure in performance probably causes an increase in anxiety. Results such as these, in which anxiety is assessed subsequent to performance, are not particularly valuable in explaining the relationship between anxiety and motor performance.

Kleine makes some methodological restrictions in order to qualify his findings. For example, he points out that up to now he has only analyzed publications in which a linear relationship between anxiety and motor performance has been reported. Curvilinear relationships, such as that present in the inverted-U function, have not yet been examined in a meta-analysis. Another reason for this, however, is that in the studies he analyzed, no test of linearity in the relationships was undertaken. A further objection lies in the fact that some of the results he reports involve dependent measurements. Nevertheless, Kleine's analysis is praiseworthy, because this is the first time that the negative relationship between anxiety and motor performance has been demonstrated using meta-analytic procedures.

Conclusions

In summary, it can be said that with regard to motoric and sport activities, anxiety research has moved from a naive-empirical approach to one that is guided by theory and strict methodology. Several developments seem particularly promising: (1) Anxiety is no longer considered a single, global construct; instead, it is analyzed with respect to its area-specific dimensions. For this reason, from the aspect of analyzing movement actions, one must also decide whether they should be interpreted in the sense of threat to self-esteem in performance tests, the risk of injury involved, whether they contain new elements unknown up to now, or whether they are carried out relatively stress- and anxiety-free to improve well-being or happiness. (2) The urgent demand to supplement cross-sectional analyses (which have long dominated research) with a process-oriented approach in empirical studies has been confronted more often in recent years. In addition to the very pragmatic assessment of the relationship between anxiety and motor performance, more studies are concentrating on the process of how anxiety originates and how it can be reduced in the context of motor-learning processes. (3) Increasing attention has been focused on the complexity of the interaction between anxiety and motor actions: not only are longitudinal studies being planned and conducted, but also preference is being given to a multilevel perspective in the choice of variables. In addition to a very careful variation of conditions regarding anxiety and stress-inducing or stress-reducing factors, multivariate operationalizations and appropriate statistical procedures are being chosen both for anxiety and movement variables. (4) The concept of meta-analysis permits a detailed, concise evaluation of different studies, above and beyond the usual review article summaries. This makes it possible to recognize current research deficits and to test possible solutions. Kleine's [1988] approach is the first attempt of this kind and deserves particular attention for this reason.

In this article we have not mentioned the subject of anxiety control and coping with anxiety. Hackfort and Schwenkmezger [1985] have summarized sport-specific theories and results concerning this topic. Krohne [1988] presents a summary of recent results in the field of high-performance sports. There is, however, a large research deficit concerning the question of whether, and under what conditions, movement actions should be used as a method of coping with anxiety situations. Topics such as which forms of movement can affect well-being or whether sport in the form of endurance training can be useful as therapy for depression have only been touched on sporadically up to now and the studies, for the most part, are methodologically weak [Schwenkmezger, 1985b].

References

Allmer, H.: Angst und Bewegungsverhalten; in Kirkcaldy, Individual differences in sport behavior, p. 224–241 (bps. Köln 1982).

Allmer, H.: Angst und Bewegungsausführung; in Rieder, Bös, Mechling, Reischle, Motorik und Bewegungsforschung, pp. 250–254 (Hofmann, Schorndorf 1983).

Ballreich, R.: Analyse und Ansteuerung sportmotorischer Techniken aus biomechanischer Sicht; in Rieder, Bös, Mechling, Reischle, Motorik und Bewegungsforschung, pp. 72–93 (Hofmann, Schorndorf 1983).

Bös, K.; Mechling, H.: Dimensionen sportmotorischer Leistungen (Hofmann, Schorndorf 1983).

Bös, K.; Mechling, H.: Bilder-Angst-Test für Bewegungssituationen (BAT). Handanweisung (Hogrefe, Göttingen 1985).

Cratty, B.J.: Motor behavior and motor learning (Lea & Febiger, Philadelphia 1967).

Deffenbacher, J.L.: Worry and emotionality in test anxiety; in Sarason, Test anxiety: Theory, research, and applications, pp. 111–128 (Erlbaum, Hillsdale 1980).

Easterbrook, J.A.: The effect of emotion on cue utilization and the organisation of behavior. Psychol. Rev. 66: 183–201 (1959).

Endler, N.S.: The interaction model of anxiety; in Landers, Christina, Psychology of motor behavior and sport – 1977, pp. 332–351 (Human Kinetics Publishers, Champaign 1978).

Eysenck, H.J.: A model for personality (Springer, New York 1981).

Eysenck, M.W.; McLeod, C.; Matthews, A.: Cognitive functioning and anxiety. Psychol. Res. *49:* 189–195 (1987).

Fahrenberg, J.; Walschburger, P.; Foerster, F.; Myrtek, M.; Müller, W.: Psychophysiologische Aktivierungsforschung. Ein Beitrag zu den Grundlagen der multivariaten Emotions- und Stress-Theorie (Minerva, München 1979).

Fiske, D.W.; Maddi, S.R.: Functions of varied experience (Dorsey Press, Homewood 1961).

Fleishman, E.A.; Hempel, W.E., Jr.: Changes in factor structure of a complex psychomotor test as a function of practice. Psychometrika *19:* 239–252 (1954).

Fröhlich, W.D.: Perspektiven der Angstforschung; in Thomae, Psychologie der Motive, Serie IV, Band 2 der Enzyklopädie der Psychologie, pp. 111–320 (Hogrefe, Göttingen 1983).

Glanzmann, P.: Anxiety, stress, and performance; in Kirkcaldy, Individual differences in movement, pp. 89–113 (MTP Press, Lancaster 1985).

Gray, J.A.: The neuropsychology of anxiety (Clarendon, Oxford 1982).

Hackfort, D.: Theorie und Diagnostik sportbezogener Ängstlichkeit; unpubl. doct. diss. DSHS Köln (1983).

Hackfort, D.; Schwenkmezger, P.: Angst und Angstkontrolle im Sport. Sportrelevante Ansätze theoretischer und empirischer Angstforschung; 2nd ed. (bps., Köln 1985).

Hackfort, D.; Schwenkmezger, P.: Measuring anxiety in sports: Possibilities, problems, and perspectives; in Spielberger, Hackfort, Anxiety in sports (Hemisphere, Washington, in press 1988).

Hodapp, V.: Causal inference from nonexperimental research on anxiety and educational achievement; in Krohne, Laux, Achievement, stress, and anxiety, pp. 355–372 (Hemisphere/Wiley, Washington 1982).

Hodapp, V.; Laux, L.; Spielberger, C.D.: Theorie und Messung der emotionalen und kognitiven Komponenten der Prüfungsangst. Different. diagnost. Psychol. *3:* 169–184 (1982).

Hollmann, W.; Hettinger, T.: Sportmedizin – Arbeits- und Trainingsgrundlagen; 2nd ed. (Schattauer, Stuttgart 1979).

Hull, C.L.: A behavior system (Yale University Press, New Haven 1952).

Hunt, V.V.; Massey, W.: Electromyographic evaluation of structural integration techniques. Psychoenergetic Systems *2:* 199–210 (1977).

Kleine, D.: Angst und sportliche Leistung; in Kunath, Proc. 7th Congr. Eur. Ass. Sport Psychol., vol. 3, pp. 882–890 (DHFK, Leipzig 1988).

Krohne, H.W.: Angsttheorie: Vom mechanistischen zum kognitiven Ansatz. Psychol. Rdsch. *31:* 12–29 (1980).

Krohne, H.W.: Coping research: Current theoretical and methodological development. Germ. J. Psychol. (in press, 1988).

Landers, D.M.: The arousal-performance relationship revisited. Res. Q. Exercise Sport *51:* 77–90 (1980).

Lazarus, R.S.; Launier, R.: Stress-related transactions between person and environment; in Pervin, Lewis, Perspectives in interactional psychology, pp. 287–327 (Plenum, New York 1978).

Liebert, R.M.; Morris, L.W.: Cognitive and emotional components of test anxiety: A distinction and some initial data. Psychol. Rep. *29:* 975–978 (1967).

Mahoney, M.J.; Avener, M.: Psychology of the elite athlete: An exploratory study. Cogn. Ther. Res. *1:* 135–141 (1977).

Martens, R.: Anxiety and motor behavior: A review. J. Motor Behav. *3:* 153–179 (1971).

Martens, R.: Arousal and motor performance; in Wilmore, Exercise and sport science review, pp. 155–188 (Wiley, New York 1974).

Martens, R.: Social psychology and physical activity (Harper & Row, New York 1975).

Martens, R.: Sport competition anxiety test (Human Kinetics Publishers, Champaign 1977).

Martens, R.: A reaction to Norman Endler's 'Interaction model of anxiety'; in Landers, Christina, Psychology of motor behavior and sport – 1977, pp. 352–358 (Human Kinetics Publishers, Champaign 1978).

Martens, R.; Landers, D.M.: Motor performance under stress: A test in reinverted – Uhypothesis. J. Pers. Soc. Psychol. *16:* 29–37 (1970).

Meinel, K.; Schnabel, G.: Bewegungslehre. Abriss einer Theorie der sportlichen Motorik unter pädagogischem Aspekt (Volkseigener Verlag, Berlin 1976).

Merrill, M.D.: Taxonomies, classifications, and theory; in Singer, The psychomotor domain: Movement behaviors, pp. 385–414 (Lea & Febiger, Philadelphia 1972).

Morris, L.W.; Davis, M.A.; Hutchings, C.A.: Cognitive and emotional components of anxiety: Literature review and a revised worry-emotionality scale. J. educ. Psychol. *73:* 541–555 (1981).

Morris, L.W.; Smith, L.R.; Andrews, E.S.; Morris, N.C.: The relationship of emotionality and worry components of anxiety to motor skills performance. J. Motor Behav. *7:* 121–130 (1975).

Myrtek, M.: Ergebnisse der psychosomatischen Korrelationsforschung. Z. Klin. Psychol. Psychother. *23:* 316–330 (1975).

Myrtek, M.: Psychophysiologische Konstitutionsforschung. Ein Beitrag zur Psychosomatik (Hogrefe, Göttingen 1982).

Nitsch, J.R.: Zur Problematik von Stressuntersuchungen; in Nitsch, Stress: Theorien, Untersuchungen, Massnahmen, pp. 142–160 (Huber, Bern 1981).

Peterson, T.: Qualitative Bewegungsforschung; in Rieder, Beiträge zur Bewegungsforschung im Sport, vol. 8 (Limpert, Bad Homburg 1985).

Poulton, E.C.: On prediction in skilled movements. Psychol. Bull. *54:* 467–478 (1957).

Sarason, I.G.: Empirical findings and theoretical problems in the use of anxiety scales. Psychol. Bull. *57:* 403–415 (1960).

Sarason, I.G.: The Test Anxiety Scale: Concepts and research; in Spielberger, Sarason, Stress and anxiety, vol. 5, pp. 193–216 (Hemisphere, Washington 1978).

Schwarzer, R.: Methodik; in Schwarzer, Meta-Analysen: Methode, Anwendungsbeispiel und Computerprogramm, pp. 1–25 (Institut für Psychologie, FU Berlin 1987).

Schwarzer, R.; Seipp, B.; Schwarzer, C.: Mathematics performance and anxiety: A meta-analysis; in Schwarzer, Meta-Analysen: Methode, Anwendungsbeispiel und Computerprogramm, pp. 26–52 (Institut für Psychologie, FU Berlin 1987).

Schwenkmezger, P.: Eigenschafts- und Zustandsangst als Prädiktoren sportspezifischer Belastung; in Genov, Proc. Vth Eur. Congr. of Sport-Psychology, vol. II, pp. 303–309 (Peoples Republic Press, Varna 1979).

Schwenkmezger, P.: Untersuchungen zur kognitiven Angsttheorie im sportmotorischen Bereich ('State-Trait-Anxiety'). Z. exp. angew. Psychol. *27:* 607–630 (1980).

Schwenkmezger, P.: Zustandsangstniveau und aufgabenfremde Kognitionen in Abhängigkeit von Trait-Angst, Erfolg und Misserfolg bei sportmotorischen Leistungen; in Michaelis, Bericht über den 32. Kongress der DGfPs in Zürich, 1980, vol. 1, pp. 354–357 (Hogrefe, Göttingen 1981).

Schwenkmezger, P.: Modelle der Eigenschafts- und Zustandsangst. Theoretische Analysen und empirische Untersuchung zur Angsttheorie von Spielberger (Hogrefe, Göttingen 1985a).

Schwenkmezger, P.: Welche Bedeutung kommt dem Ausdauertraining in der Depressionstherapie zu? Sportwissenschaft *15:* 117–135 (1985b).

Schwenkmezger, P.; Laux, L.: Trait anxiety, worry, and emotionality in athletic competition; in Spielberger, Diaz-Guerrero, Cross-cultural anxiety, vol. 3, pp. 65–77 (Hemisphere, Washington 1986).

Singer, R.; Ungerer-Röhrich, U.: Vergleichende Untersuchungen zur Validität allgemeiner und sportpsychologischer Angsttests; in Schilling, Herren, Bericht zum VI. FEPSAC-Kongress 1983, vol. 1, pp. 117–123 (ETS, Magglingen 1985).

Sonstroem, R.J.; Bernardo, P.: Interindividual pregame state anxiety and basketball performance: A reexamination of the inverted U-curve. J. Sport Psychol. *4:* 235–245 (1982).

Späte, D.; Schwenkmezger, P.: Leistungsbestimmende psychische Merkmale bei Handballspielern. Leistungssport *13:* 11–19 (1983).

Spence, J.T.; Spence, K.W.: The motivational components of manifest anxiety: Drive and drive stimuli; in Spielberger, Anxiety and behavior, pp. 291–326 (Academic Press, New York 1966).

Spence, K.W.: A theory of emotionally based drive (D) and its relation to performance in simple learning situations. Am. Psychol. *13:* 131–141 (1958).

Spielberger, C.D.: Theory and research in anxiety; in Spielberger, Anxiety and behavior, pp. 3–20 (Academic Press, New York 1966).

Spielberger, C.D.: Anxiety as an emotional state; in Spielberger, Anxiety: Current trends in theory and research, vol. 1, pp. 23–49 (Academic Press, New York 1972).

Spielberger, C.D.; Gorsuch, R.L.; Lushene, R.E.: STAI: Manual for the State-Trait-Anxiety Inventory (Consulting Psychologist Press, Palo Alto 1970).

Taylor, J.A.: A personality scale of manifest anxiety. J. abnorm. soc. Psychol. *48:* 285–290 (1953).

Taylor, J.A.: Drive theory and manifest anxiety. Psychol. Bull. *53:* 303–320 (1956).

Weinberg, R.S.: Anxiety and motor behavior: A new direction; in Christina, Landers, Psychology of motor behavior and sport – 1976, vol. II, pp. 132–139 (Human Kinetics Publishers, Champaign 1977).

Weinberg, R.S.: The effects of success and failure on the patterning of neuromuscular energy. J. Motor Behav. *10:* 53–61 (1978).

Weinberg, R.S.: Anxiety and motor performance: Drive theory vs. cognitive theory. Int. J. Sport Psychol. *10:* 112–121 (1979).

Weinberg, R.S.; Hunt, V.V.: The interrelationships between anxiety, motor performance, and electromyography. J. Motor Behav. *8:* 219–224 (1976).

Weinberg, R.S.; Ragan, J.: Motor performance under three levels of trait anxiety and stress. J. Motor Behav. *10:* 169–176 (1978).

Wine, J.D.: Test anxiety and direction of attention. Psychol. Bull. *76:* 92–104 (1971).

Wine, J.D.: Cognitive-attentional theory of test anxiety; in Sarason, Test anxiety: Theory, research and applications, pp. 349–385 (Erlbaum, Hillsdale 1980).

Wine, J.D.: Evaluation anxiety: A cognitive attentional construct; in Krohne, Laux, Achievement, stress, and anxiety, pp. 207–219 (Hemisphere/Wiley, Washington 1982).

Yerkes, R.M.; Dodson, J.D.: The relationship of strength of stimulus to rapidity of habit formation. J. comp. Neurol. Psychol. *18:* 459–482 (1908).

Peter Schwenkmezger, PhD, Fachbereich I Psychologie, Postfach 3825, Universität Trier, D–5500 Trier (FRG)

Kirkcaldy B (ed): Normalities and Abnormalities in Human Movement.
Med Sport Sci. Basel, Karger, 1989, vol 29, pp 100–127

Motor Abnormalities and the Psychopathology of Schizophrenia[1]

Theo C. Manschreck

Experimental Psychopathology, Massachusetts General Hospital,
Harvard Medical School, Boston, Mass., USA

Introduction

Motor abnormalities in schizophrenia, often neglected in the past, are now the focus of considerable research and clinical interest. They include a spectrum of voluntary and involuntary disturbances of varying frequency and severity, affecting such features as gait, general movement, and intentional action.

As a rule, they have been difficult to study because of a lack of guiding hypotheses and effective measures, their fluctuating nature, and, to be sure, a reluctance to interpret their occurrence in terms of brain dysfunction. Yet, they have been observed repeatedly and long before the development of modern pharmacologic therapies. Dramatic features like catalepsy, posturing, and excitement and more common, often subtle, ones like stereotypies, mannerisms, clumsiness, and incoordination have been described for years [1–4]. Beyond classification and description, however, we know little about them, and there have been remarkably few studies to change that circumstance. Despite extensive commentary on motor behavior in schizophrenia, no systematic explanation has been put forward, nor have there been many attempts to evaluate the relationship of motor features with other classes of symptoms – both of which seem essential to a satisfactory account of schizophrenia.

The study of motor disturbances could permit relating of observable, measurable behavior to other aspects of brain function and anatomy such

[1] Much of this chapter was previously published in the Handbook of Schizophrenia, vol. 1: The Neurology of Schizophrenia (Elsevier, Amsterdam 1986).

that localization of pathology may become possible. This potential contrasts with the limitations that plague the assessment of delusional, hallucinatory, and other subjective disturbances of schizophrenic illness. Indeed a clearer understanding of the neurology of schizophrenic motor behavior holds the promise of advances in differential diagnosis, etiology, pathogenesis, and treatment. This chapter presents a summary of described motor abnormalities of schizophrenia, and reviews relevant clinical, high risk, and laboratory studies. While our understanding of the neurology of such abnormalities is limited, this knowledge provides a foundation and direction for further development.

Motor Features of Schizophrenia

Although there is little specific knowledge about motor features in schizophrenia, they have been consistently observed in remarkable variety over the years. Despite the current confounding factor of antipsychotic drug treatment in most modern cases, their discovery clearly precedes the use of chlorpromazine [1, 2, 5]. Attempts to classify them must, to some extent, be arbitrary. The scheme used here divides examples of reported abnormal behavior, regardless of specificity, frequency, or uniqueness to schizophrenia into those associated with increased movement (hyperkinesia) those associated with decreased movement (hypokinesia) compared to normal behavior. These categories are then subdivided according to whether the feature is diffuse or patterned. The disturbances associated with diminished motor activity in schizophrenia encompass retardation, poverty of movement, and stupor *(diffuse)*, and motor blocking (obstruction), cooperation, opposition (gegenhalten), automatic obedience, negativism, ambitendency, echopraxia, and last-minute responses *(patterned)*. In contrast, disturbances related to increased motor activity in schizophrenia include 'diffuse' features such as restlessness, excitement, tremor, stereotyped movements (stereotypies), spasms, choreiform movements, athetoid movements, parakinesia, myoclonic movements, perseverative movements, impulsive movements, carphologic movements, agitation, tics and mannerisms. Disorders of posture [6] are usually considered a form of motor disturbance (increased muscle tonus in isolated areas of the body, manneristic postures, stereotyped postures, waxy flexibility, and clumsiness). The features of catatonia, a classic syndrome of motor disturbance, overlap several of these categories. Although it is sometimes difficult in practice to distinguish drug-induced effects from those associated with psychiatric illness itself, both have distinct characteristics.

Early Observations

Kraepelin's [2] description of the motor features, of dementia praecox, emphasized their intermittent, variable, subtle, and occasionally dramatic nature. Among patients with diagnoses of dementia praecox, Kraepelin noted multiple motor features, including echopraxia, catalepsy, forms of negativism, stupor, and reduced efficiency of fine movements. A marked clumsiness, jerkiness, or loss of smooth muscular coordination also characterized these patients. Kraepelin described the gait of the patient as having the appearance of walking through snow. Although the catatonic subtype of dementia praecox was dominated by motor disturbance features, Kraepelin observed similar features in the hebephrenic and paranoid forms of the disorder as well. Kraepelin discovered that motor efficiency in a specific task deteriorated rapidly. In handiwork and crafts, particularly those involving fine work, he and others noted a general decline in ability [7, 8]. Kraepelin also recognized that movement disorders suggestive of dementia praecox could be the consequence of known neurological diseases including encephalitis, syphilis, and epilepsy, and he emphasized the value of differential diagnosis and careful follow-up to sort out such alternative explanations.

Bleuler [5] described many of the same motor features that Kraepelin had identified among dementia praecox patients, noting that motor anomalies were seldom absent. He also commented on 'idiomuscular contractions', spasms, and a 'will 'o the wisp' gait, with irregular timing and spacing of steps.

Although his ideas concerning the hierarchical organization of the central nervous system derived from the study of neurological disease, Jackson [9] considered his concepts applicable to mental disorders. In mental illness, he maintained, there is a dissolution of the highest cerebral centers. Complex functions normally under voluntary control are lost. Consequently, less complex and undamaged central nervous system components produce the striking manifestations of mental disorder.

Jackson proposed that, in psychosis, clinical features can be classified according to whether they result from dissolution (so-called negative symptoms) or from activity in the remaining undamaged nervous components (so-called positive symptoms). Negative symptoms of schizophrenia would include withdrawal, blocking, disturbances of identity, and passivity experiences. Positive symptoms would include hallucinations, delusions, stereotypies, mannerisms, and catalepsy.

Similar views were put forward by Carl Wernicke and Karl Kahlbaum who argued that focal cerebral pathology was the basis for the motor features of psychotic disorders. The idea that subcortical mechanisms produce these features when deprived of the influence of higher centers has been popular. Kleist [1], for example, felt that schizophrenic motor disturbances had a source identical to that of neurological disease with similar motor manifestations. Other writers have echoed this theme [4, 10–12].

Jaspers [13] noted certain remarkable characteristics of schizophrenic motor features. For instance, while there is increased muscle tone in certain limbs or areas, such as the face of a patient maintaining a catatonic posture, there is decreased or normal tone in other areas of the body, a kind of incoordination or fragmentation of motor function. Jaspers also observed that the 'immobile' catatonic patient could initiate such basic activities as care of toileting, feeding, and dressing but was often unable to respond to verbal requests.

Jaspers coined the term psychomotor disturbance and applied it to schizophrenia to suggest that the similarity between schizophrenic motor features and the features of certain neurological syndromes did not necessarily reflect a common set of causes or pathogenesis [14]. In catatonic excitement, on the other hand, patients may identify with their behavior and attempt to construct rationalizations for it. When outwardly similar behavior occurs in encephalitis lethargica, for example, patients tend to be distressed, bewildered, occasionally confused by their motor symptoms.

Freeman [15] also compared the clinical motor phenomena characteristic of chronic schizophrenia and those characteristic of organic mental disorder. In schizophrenia, particularly the catatonic and hebephrenic subtypes, disturbances in such voluntary movements as blocking, overly repetitive activity, and difficulty in switching to new movements can be observed frequently in spontaneous behavior and elicited on examination (e.g., using Luria's tests of motility). Disturbed movement is more likely to occur when the patient is inattentive, distractible, and generally unresponsive. The same characteristics are frequently found in other organic conditions although the appearance of normal motility is rare in progressive degenerative disease. Even in schizophrenia, Freeman argues, normal motility is uncommon. The movements that recur in so-called normal fashion in schizophrenia are those that could be described as highly practiced.

The promising potential of these early observations was not realized because of the widespread view that motor features are secondary to more primary psychological disturbances; a paucity of useful performance measures for reliably defining the motor capacities of schizophrenic patients; the inconsistent nature of motor disturbances, which suggests they are not essential characteristics, and fundamentally, the absence of a model that could predict and explain the relationships among thought, will, emotion, and motor anomalies [16]. The probability that schizophrenia is a heterogeneous group of disorders has also provided a methodological barrier to rapid progress in the study of motor anomaly. The following sections summarize the variety and complexity of motor abnormalities in schizophrenia and indicate some of the gaps in our knowledge.

Catatonia and Catatonic Schizophrenia

Although Kahlbaum [17], as well as Kraepelin and Bleuler, stressed that catatonic behavior has a number of different possible etiologies, there has been a tendency to regard catatonic behavior as signifying schizophrenia. It is, of course, well known that fluorides, hyperparathyroidism, viral encephalitides, manic-depressive disorder, tuberculosis, and other diseases can be the source of catatonic behavior [18]. Indeed, immobility, stupor, catalepsy, posturing, grimacing, stereotyping behavior, and negativism – that is, catatonia – constitute a syndrome that has been described in numerous psychiatric and medical disorders. Classically, there are two extreme patterns of catatonic behavior – a retarded or withdrawn stupor, and a hyperkinetic, occasionally aggressive, excitement.

Kraepelin believed that, when these patterns were persistent, not diagnosable as part of known disease, and associated with disturbances of will, judgment, and emotion, they formed a subtype of dementia praecox. Slater and Roth [14] claim, as do others, that the more prevalent type of catatonic behavior in schizophrenia is retarded or withdrawn. And certainly, catatonic schizophrenia has been associated with the most obvious and dramatic motor disturbances. Yet motor anomalies of schizophrenia are not limited to this subtype. As Kraepelin and Bleuler both observed, motor disturbances occur in all subtypes of schizophrenia. When motor disturbances predominate, most cases are diagnosed catatonic. When motor disturbances are not detectable, or less striking, other characteristics (e.g., thought disturbance or paranoid thinking) have tended to determine subtype classification.

Matters are considerably less clear in contemporary clinical settings. Most schizophrenic patients manifest a mixture of catatonic, hebephrenic, and paranoid features, and few qualify for the classic subtype labels. This circumstance has resulted in the increased diagnosis of undifferentiated schizophrenia. Indeed, there has been a reduction in the diagnosis of catatonic and hebephrenic subtypes over the last 50 years, although the overall prevalence (about 1 %) of schizophrenia appears to be stable [19]. For instance, it is increasingly uncommon to find obvious catatonic slowing, rigidity, or related classic features. When they do occur, they usually are short lived, often subtle, and frequently not associated with schizophrenic disorder [20, 21].

Some [22, 23] have suggested that certain neurological disorders with varied epidemiologic patterns (e.g., encephalitis of Parkinson's disease) may have contributed to such changes. Others [24] have documented patterns of assigning the catatonic subtype diagnosis that indicate poor reliability. Whatever the source, shifts in the incidence of symptoms and signs make more difficult attempts to determine the frequency and nature of motor features in schizophrenia.

Not surprisingly, knowledge of incidence, prevalence, and natural history of motor features is sketchy because few reliable estimates appear in either the older or more recent literature [4, 25]. Much of the relevant information concerns specific motor anomalies, such as stereotypies, as discussed below.

Specific Motor Abnormalities

Descriptive studies of specific abnormal movements such as stereotypies, are complicated by problems of definition and interpretation. Lacking standard terminology, investigators have relied on their own concepts. Generally, only major or clinically obvious manifestations have been examined. Little work has attempted to explore more subtle features, such as clumsiness or incoordination, or the impact of motor disturbance on skilled performance [26]. Most investigators have failed to assess these anomalies longitudinally.

The incidence and prevalence of choreiform and athetoid movements in psychiatric patients remains somewhat controversial. Mettler and Crandell [27] estimated that choreiform movements occurred frequently among schizophrenic patients and especially among chronic patients in psychiatric hospitals. Others [4], however, have claimed that these movements occur in neurological disease, especially of the basal ganglia, and should not be considered part of the schizophrenic syndrome. Their frequent occurrence in tardive dyskinesia would tend to support this argument.

Perseveration is a well-known clinical sign of disturbed motor and speech behavior among neurologically and psychiatrically disordered individuals. Allison [28] documented that perseveration occurs in a wide variety of conditions.

Freeman and Gathercole [29] examined perseveration in chronic schizophrenia and dementia. Extensive testing using a number of methods to elicit forms of perseverative behavior was undertaken in a group of schizophrenic and demented patients. The result provided no evidence for a unitary trait of perseveration.

Knowledge of echopraxia and echolalia has progressed in limited ways. Stengel [30] showed that echo reactions were common in a number of different conditions, although they have been considered a classic feature of catatonic disorder. Transcortical aphasia, mental deficiency, chronic epilepsy, delirium, early speech development in children, and states of fatigue and inattention in normals were the main disorders associated with echo phenomena. Echo phenomena tended to be associated in these conditions with an urge to act or speak, a tendency to repetition, and incomplete development or impairment in perception and expression of speech.

Jones and Hunter [25] reported a 2-year longitudinal study of abnormal movements in a group of chronic institutionalized psychiatric patients, one-third of whom had not received antipsychotic medication. Of the 127, 87% were diagnosed as schizophrenics. Approximately 25% of the entire sample had diagnosed brain disorder and/or subnormal intelligence, although this group was not separated from the larger group in reporting observations. The investigators looked at four kinds of movements: tremor, choreoathetosis, tics, and stereotypies (by which they mean any form of movements, apart from the other categories, that became abnormal because of repetition).

The authors concluded that there is a high incidence and variability in patterns of abnormal movements among long-stay psychiatric patients. Tics, stereotypies, and choreoathetosis occurred more frequently in those who at some time had received antipsychotic medication. However, examination of records disclosed that abnormal movements of all types had been present in patients never treated with neuroleptics. In some patients, abnormal movements developed only after years of exposure to drugs; in others, only after drugs had been discontinued for months. Choreoathetosis, though least common, was the most persistent. Its occurrence in older patients as well as its association with neurological impairment suggest that it is not typically part of schizophrenia. Tics, tremors, and stereotypies tended to occur transiently, although continuous patterns of stereotypy were also evident. Episodes of restlessness, nowadays usually associated with neuroleptic treatment, were common in the early stages of mental disorder and recurred in some patients over many years, independent of treatment.

This report was one of the few systematic attempts to evaluate the incidence and natural history of reported motor disturbances in schizophrenia. The inclusion of patients with known organic impairment makes interpretation difficult because motor anomalies are common in brain disease. Moreover, the study failed to examine the full range of motor abnormalities in schizophrenia. Nevertheless, the findings clearly indicate that motor disturbances occur frequently, variably, and usually subtly in schizophrenia.

A British study [31] has examined spontaneous involuntary disorders of movement in a sample of 411 hospitalized patients with chronic schizophrenia [32]. The findings, based on standardized rating techniques, the Abnormal Involuntary Movement Scale (AIMS) and the more detailed Rockland Scale, indicated a high prevalence of involuntary movement abnormalities in the sample. With at least moderate degrees of severity, 50.6% of the patients had demonstrable anomalies of one or more of AIMS items; the corresponding Rockland Scale figure was 67.6%. The major component of abnormality was contributed by rating of facial movements. Of particular interest was the opportunity to assess a subsample of 47 patients with no history of exposure to neuroleptic drugs. The authors found no differences in the prevalence and severity of movement disturbances and few differences in regional distribution of abnormality. They concluded that spontaneous involuntary movements can be a feature of chronic schizophrenia that is unmodified by drugs.

The study unfortunately did not report on disturbances in voluntary patterns of movement disorder. Assessment of neurological abnormalities resulted in relatively few, generally minor peripheral findings. An important additional observation was that the movements considered in the study exhibited considerable stability in gross distribution and severity during a 12- to 18-month period of follow-up.

Onset and Relationship to Prognosis

No one knows precisely when abnormal movements have their onset in schizophrenia (see High-Risk Studies section), but motor manifestations typically have been reported to occur after the appearance of other symptoms. Schneider [33] offered an approach to diagnosis of schizophrenia in its early stages, in part because dramatic observable motor disturbances in acute cases are uncommon. His first-rank symptoms reflect subjective experiences of an unusual and incomprehensible sort from the standpoint of normal human experience. Auditory hallucinations, delusional perception, and several forms of passivity experience constitute the symptoms that Schneider believed were pathognomonic for acute schizophrenia, if coarse brain disease was not present. Two of the passivity experiences (i.e., made impulses, made acts) suggest disturbance affecting motor functions, and reflect a sense of loss of control and coordination of movement not necessarily discernible to others. While the claim to pathognomonicity has been criticized [34–36], there is general agreement that first-rank symptoms are highly discriminating symptoms for the diagnosis of schizophrenic disorder.

In 1966, Chapman [37] coined the term 'ideokinetic apraxia' to describe the difficulties in sequential motor activities (e.g. walking, eating, and sitting down) reported by patients early in the course of illness. Movements seemed slow, required more deliberation and concentration, and felt more restricted than normal. Patients described a loss of automaticity of movements and a heightened awareness of bodily processes. In 33% of patients, motor and thought blocking characterized by transient immobility, blank expression, and fixed gaze were common. Echolalia and echopraxia also occurred in some cases. For 33%, mutism was encountered at some point during the course of illness. In some patients, prolonged catatonic behavior and gross visual perceptual disturbances were associated with a deteriorating course.

These findings raise the possibility that objective assessment techniques, such as motor performance tests, might succeed in detecting early motor difficulties. Subjective accounts are helpful, but objective means would be more satisfactory to extend our knowledge of the natural history of motor phenomena in schizophrenia.

The relationship between prognosis and motor disturbance is unclear. Kraepelin [2], of course, believed that dementia praecox has a poor outcome. He and Bleuler both noted that stereotypic movements could persist for many years, and eventually become progressively more simplified, but preoccupying nonetheless, occurring independent of apparent expressive purpose. They often were associated with verbigeration of thought disorder [1]. And many maintain that motor disturbances such as stereotypies that may occur early in the course of schizophrenia portend a poor prognosis. There have been few studies to confirm or refute such opinions. Jones [38] found no relationship between complexity of stereotypies and age of onset, length of illness, or duration of hospitalization in 13 chronic schizophrenics with stereotypic behavior.

Yarden and Discipio [39] investigated the idea that an earlier onset of movement disorder is associated with poor prognosis. The movements were primarily choreiform and athetoid, but included tics, stereotypies, and mannerisms. The patients were described as free of neurological disease, retardation, or history of chronic hospitalization. These patients, compared to a control group of schizophrenics without abnormal movements, had an earlier age of onset of changes in mental state and longer hospitalizations. Patients with abnormal movements also showed significantly more severe thought disorder, purposeless activity, negativism, and neglect of personal hygiene. This group was less affected than the control group by pharmacologic interventions. Moreover, the presence of abnormal movements was associated with a significantly poorer prognosis for the period of study.

An Investigation of Motor Movements in Schizophrenic Disorders

Manschreck et al. [3] investigated the occurrence of the classic reported motor disturbances in schizophrenics and their relationship to other features of the illness. Subtype diagnosis, affective blunting, neurological nonlocalizing signs, delusions, and formal thought disorder were of particular interest.

Thirty-seven patients were examined who met the DSM III criteria for the diagnosis of schizophrenic disorders, including paranoid, disorganized, undifferentiated, and catatonic types. The affective disorder group totaled 16 and consisted of manic, schizoaffective (manic type), schizoaffective (depressed disorder), and psychotic depressives. These groups did not differ by age, education, length of illness, or neuroleptic drug treatment.

The assessment included ratings of spontaneous behavior and behavior elicited by the examiner (shake your head, open and then close your eyes, clap your hands three times. Ozeretski's test, fist-ring test, fist-edge-palm test, station and gait, tests of coordination, such as rapid alternating movements and finger-nose-finger-test). Disturbances in voluntary motor behavior were detectable in all but one schizophrenic (subtype paranoid) and were infrequent among affective subjects, except for the schizoaffective subtype. The most common form of spontaneous motor abnormality in schizophrenics was clumsiness or awkwardness, a postural disturbance. The second most common were stereotypic and manneristic movements followed by motor blocking. Not observed in this sample were ambitendency, catalepsy, automatic obedience, choreoathetoid movements, excitement, and stupor. Of the subtypes, a smaller proportion of the paranoid group exhibited spontaneous motor abnormalities (31%), whereas all of the disorganized (hebephrenic) subjects showed such anomalies.

On the other hand, with the exception of the schizoaffective group, the performance of affective subjects was generally normal. Indeed, 4 of the 5 schizoaffective subjects exhibited at least one feature of abnormal motor behavior on examination. (The effect of antipsychotic medication on movements was examined. The results suggest that neuroleptics tend to reduce the number and/or severity of such abnormalities.)

There was a positive and significant association between motor features and affective blunting and between nonlocalizing neurological signs and motor features. But the most striking association was the one between total abnormal intrinsic motor features and formal disturbances of thinking ($r = 0.62$, $p < 0.001$, one-tailed). There was no evidence of a relationship between voluntary motor disturbances and delusional thinking.

In summary, the main finding was that disturbances in voluntary motor behavior (i.e., those that were not attributable to drug effects or known neurological disorder) occur in virtually all cases of conservatively defined schizophrenic disorder. The observed abnormalities were generally short-lived phenomena that might easily be missed if they were not carefully scrutinized. The fact that additional procedures for eliciting motor disturbance increased the number of observed abnormalities indicates that routine examination of occasional observation may not detect their presence. Indeed, the optimal method for discovering motor disturbances is clinical observation of patients over extended periods. Notably, the techniques for examination overlap only somewhat with the standard neurological examination.

It is also worth noting that certain dramatic features were not in evidence (e.g., automatic obedience, catalepsy, or excitement). And only 1 of the 37 schizophrenics qualified for the subtype diagnosis of catatonia. These observations are consistent with current reports of reduced incidence of catatonic schizophrenia. Yet abnormal movements were ubiquitous among the schizophrenic subjects regardless of subtype, tempting the suggestion that they have been neglected largely because the search for motor manifestations has been focused on fairly uncommon and unusual features to the exclusion of more common ones [40].

The relative absence of motor disturbances in affective subjects suggests that while these features are certainly not pathognomonic for schizophrenia, they tend to be significantly concentrated among individuals bearing that diagnosis. Of considerable interest is the fact that it was among the schizoaffective subgroup of affective subjects (a grouping that is controversial based on the presence of both schizophrenic and affective features) that most of the voluntary motor disturbances occurred.

The fact that affective blunting and nonlocalizing neurological signs also were associated with disturbed motor features points to interesting implications. The latter features have been considered evidence for subtle neurological impairment in schizophrenia. The frequency of affective blunting and neurological sign incidence is also consistent with published reports [41].

A second finding of the study was the significant, positive association of motor abnormality and disturbance in the form of thinking. The coincidence among schizophrenics of features from both these dimensions of behavioral functioning suggests that they may have a common pathogenetic basis.

The potentially difficult problem of neuroleptic drug effects was dealt with by the careful measurement of drug-induced motor activity and its exclusion from the computation of the motor behavior abnormality that was related to thought disorder. The incidence of neuroleptic side effects was consistent with previous reports and thus argues against a systematic underestimation of such effects. Moreover, we found significant differences between disturbed voluntary movement scores of medicated and nonmedicated schizophrenics, suggesting that drugs tend to reduce those anomalies. On the other hand, in the paired comparisons of medicated schizophrenic and affective subjects, schizophrenic patients had significantly more voluntary motor disturbances, suggesting that motor impairment is more closely associated with the latter disorder.

It is naturally possible that some drug effects not detected by the rating scale methods we employed might be present (while other dramatic extrapyramidal features were absent), which could interfere with the programmed sequence of motor acts and the initiation of voluntary motor activity. The elicited motor activity assessments would be most susceptible to such effects; a separate analysis of the schizophrenic motor features observed in spontaneous behavior and formal thought disorder proved consistent with the hypothesized relationship between language and motor disturbance.

High-Risk Studies

Information is limited regarding the natural history of motor abnormalities. While follow-up studies will undoubtedly augment our knowledge, evidence from high-risk studies makes an important contribution.

Fish [42] reports that motor symptoms are often found in children who suffer psychiatric disturbance at a later age. For example, Robins [43, 44] observed the difficulty walking differentiated preschizophrenic children from others. Watt [45] found that neurological disturbance and severe organic handicaps were more common at an earlier age among children who later developed schizophrenia than among classroom controls. Ricks and Nameche [46] discovered slow motor development and nonspecific neurological symptoms twice as often in preschizophrenics as in controls, and more frequently in the group that became chronically disordered compared to that which experienced a more benign course of schizophrenia [47]. Such prominent symptoms as hyperactivity, rigidity, abnormal gait, poor coordination, and impaired attention were typical among those who later became chronically withdrawn schizophrenics.

Marcus [48] investigated so-called neurological soft signs in a group of 7- to 14-year-olds born of schizophrenic parents and a group of matched controls whose parents had no mental disease. He determined that facial asymmetry, fine motor coordination, left-right orientation, and evidence of disturbances of visual perception and auditory-visual integration were significantly more common among the high-risk sample. In the obstetric studies of high-risk individuals, conducted by Mednick et al. [49] retarded motor development at 5 days and 1 year differentiated offspring of schizophrenics from controls. Dozenko and Fatovi [cf. 42], using Ozeretski's method of studying motor maturity of children of schizophrenics, found that disturbances in speed, simultaneous movements, time and rhythm were the maximally decreased skills of motor function that distinguished the high-risk children. Fish's own work on infants at risk shows a spectrum of mild to severe irregularities and disruptions of physical growth as well as gross motor and visual-motor developmental abnormalities. These anomalies are associated with the later development of a spectrum of psychiatric disturbances. The presence of developmental disorders and complications thereof were significantly related to being at genetic risk for schizophrenia and not to pregnancy and birth complication history.

Hanson et al. [50] completed a study of children of schizophrenic parents. At age 4, 30% of these children demonstrated poor motor skills in hopping, walking a line, catching a ball, and finer tasks, such as stringing beads. Three variables – poor motor skills, the presence of large intraindividual inconsistency of performance in various cognitive tasks, and observations of apathy, withdrawal, flatness, instability of relationships, irritability, and negativism – were chosen as predictors of vulnerability to schizophrenia on the basis of previous reports. These variables at extreme thresholds characterized 5 of 116 children, an incidence of about 10 times chance expectation. These 5 were all offspring of schizophrenic parents, and their case histories showed enduring forms of maladjustment of the types reported in the premorbid history of schizophrenia. In another longitudinal study [51] evidence of premorbid neuromotor deviancies (e.g. poor gross and fine motor abilities) has also been associated with vulnerability to psychopathology among high-risk adolescents.

In sum, studies of high-risk populations suggest that motor development delays and impairment of motor abilities, especially fine motor coordination, are detectable at an early age and may be associated with later development of schizophrenia, possibly of a more severe form.

Additional Studies

The findings of the investigation of motor abnormalities in schizophrenic disorder reported above led to two additional studies [52, 53]. In the first, focus was set on the relationship between formal thought disorder and clinical motor disturbance with more objective measures of language disorganization. In the second, a laboratory measure was developed of motor function, to compare disorganization on motor performance among schizophrenic and control subjects with assessments of thinking and motor behavior.

In the first study, we decided to measure the type-token ratio (TTR) because it is a simple, reliable, and quantifiable index of language deviance, unbiased by clinical judgment, and because in prior reports the TTR as an index of spoken language disorganization is statistically lower for formal thought-disordered schizophrenics compared to nonthought-disordered schizophrenics and psychiatric controls [52]. Also age, education, and medication status do not appear to substantially influence this difference. The TTR is a measure of variability (or repetitiousness) in lexicon usage and is computed by dividing the total number of words (tokens into the number of different words (types) in samples of uniform length).

Thus, the first study extending the survey examined the hypothesis that disruptions in language behavior, as indicated by the TTR, would be associated with clinical evidence of disruptions in motor movement. Samples of language (at least 100 words) assessed using the mean segmental type-token ratio (MSTTR) measure, which represents the average of TTRs for consecutive segments of 100 words. The motor response testing was the same as described in the survey study.

The subjects included 21 schizophrenics (10 with evidence of formal thought disorder – 5 disorganized and 5 undifferentiated phenomenological subtypes). The 11 nonthought-disordered schizophrenics included 8 paranoid and 3 undifferentiated subtypes. There were 12 affective subjects (6 major depressives, 3 manics, and 3 schizoaffectives, manic type) and 12 normals. None of the affective or normal controls had clinical evidence of formal thought disorder.

Each schizophrenic and several affective subjects (schizoaffective types, in particular) showed evidence of disruption of skilled motor performance in the testing procedure. The relationship between scores summarizing evidence of disruption in skilled motor movements and MSTTRs was analyzed and the results indicated a negative association ($r = -0.59$, d.f. $= 32$, $p < 0.001$).

The main finding then was that indices of disorganized motor behavior and language are strongly associated. Age and education appear to have little impact on the basic correlation. This point to a potentially important relationship between disruptions in speech and movements behavior especially in, but not limited to, schizophrenics, particularly among the thought-disordered subgroup. The use of an index of language disturbance, the TTR, more reliable than the usual clinical ratings, represents an extension of and further support for the association between formal thought disorder and disrupted movements, a feature of schizophrenia not confounded by language.

This study also pointed to the need for assessments of motor behavior that would be free of the inherent bias of clinical evaluation techniques in order to complement the greater reliability of language measures, such as the TTR.

The laboratory study of motor deficit [53] in schizophrenic disorders poses two problems: one is to establish that a reliable relationship exists between clinically observed motor phenomena and laboratory measures of the deficit; the second is to establish that the motor anomalies have a reliable relationship with some other important aspect of the psychopathological syndrome, including evidence of structural or physiologic change.

Workers investigating the components of skilled motor performance have made extensive use of the concept of redundancy. From the standpoint of information theory, any event can be regarded as redundant to the extent that it is predictable from observation of a chain of immediately prior events. An object moving through space with fixed course and velocity is moving with high redundancy, whereas an insect flitting unpredictably from one point to another is moving with low redundancy. Simple rhythmic movements, such as are seen in the repeated hammering of a nail or the polishing of a surface, are examples of high-redundancy activities. Such patterns of motor activity permit adaptive responsiveness to other stimuli in the environment. Where an individual is deficient in the adaptive use of redundancies, we should expect rhythmic performance to be impaired. Indeed, some investigations reported elsewhere suggest that this is the case [54, 55].

There is substantial evidence that schizophrenic patients fail to make use of redundancy [56] and that this is associated with the presence of thought disorder in these patients [57, 58]. On this basis it seems reasonable to study rhythmic behavior in schizophrenic patients. We predicted that schizophrenics would be less able than nonschizophrenic controls to synchronize a motor movement with rhythmic stimuli. However, defective performance among schizophrenic patients on almost any task is practically axiomatic. Hence, it was necessary to be sure that by varying the difficulty of the rhythm task it would be possible to detect differential deficit in the performance of schizophrenic subjects and not a uniform depression of adequacy of response across all conditions. We also expected that those patients who showed the most marked deficit would show deficits in the nonmotor sphere (i.e. in thought disorder).

We decided to select rates of response that ranged from too low to permit accuracy to too high to do so. In this respect the investigation offered the possibility of establishing the task limits that would serve to detect differential deficit in schizophrenic and other psychiatric patients.

We hypothesized that (a) schizophrenic performance on a rhythm synchronization task would reflect a relative incapacity to automate a motor performance (i.e., to rhythmize repetitive motor behavior) and would not be explainable by task difficulty; (b) clinical evidence of motor disturbance would be associated with evidence of poorer relative performance of the laboratory, and (c) laboratory motor abnormality would be associated with severity of formal thought disorder.

Subjects were selected by strict diagnostic criteria [32] and by Research Diagnostic Criteria (RDC) [59]. Sixteen schizophrenics were studied, including 5 paranoid, 7 disorganized, and 4 undifferentiated subtypes. Eight normal and 8 psychiatric (affective psychosis) controls were studied, including 5 major depressives and 3 schizoaffectives. Eleven of 16 schizophrenic subjects and 6 of 8 affective controls were taking neuroleptic medication. Dosages were matched according to chlorpromazine equivalents.

The procedure for clinical assessments of motor, thinking, and neuroleptic effects followed that of the survey investigation. Language samples were also obtained for TTR assessment of language disorganization. The synchronization task took place in a quiet, windowless laboratory. An Ester-line Angus variable speed signal generator was used to produce rhythmic stimuli – uniform acoustic clicks. Unaccented (i.e., uniform) clicks create what is called a tremolo rhythmic pattern [60]. For each trial, randomly ordered series of standard volume acoustic clicks of one rate (8, 12, 20, 40, 80, 120, 200, or 400 beats/min) was presented. A wide range of rates was employed because it was not clear at which one the predictability of clicks would influence performance; although it was thought likely that at extreme-ly slow and fast rates, this factor would exert less influence on accuracy, than the ability to estimate intervals and tapping speed, respectively. To ensure that the effects of change in the rate were not confounded by changes in the pattern of rhythm, only the rate of clicks varied across trials. Synchroniza-tion was defined as simultaneous stimulus and subject response.

To determine the extent of the relationship between clinical and labora-tory findings, the following strategy was applied. Disturbed motor activity scores, formal thought disturbance, and type-token ratios were compared among all subjects with synchronization accuracy at the rate that most distinguished the subject groups.

The results of this study can be summarized as follows. First, 15 of 16 schizophrenic subjects manifested one or more of the features of formal thought disorder, while 3 of the psychiatric controls showed such distur-bance. Second, clinical motor disturbances were evident among all but 2 schizophrenics, whereas only 3 psychiatric controls showed such evidence. Normal controls showed no evidence of thought or motor abnormality. Third, evidence of neuroleptic side effects occurred in 2 (25%) of the 8 affective psychotic controls and in 5 (45%) of the 11 schizophrenic subjects taking neuroleptics. Within each group, subjects with neuroleptic side effects did not differ from those without side effects on ratings of other disturbed motor behavior. Medicated [11] and nonmedicated [5] schizophrenic subjects did not differ in clinical motor ratings. On the other hand, medicated schi-zophrenic subjects and medicated affective controls were significantly differ-ent in clinical motor ratings (t(14) = 3.05, p < 0.005).

Fourth, our initial hypothesis – that schizophrenic group performance would be distinctive and not explained by task difficulty – was supported. The schizophrenic group was as able as normal or psychiatric control groups to rhythmize (or synchronize) performance at the slower rates (i.e., at 40 beats/min or slower) and at the faster rate of 200 beats/min. This suggests that difficulty cannot account for these results and that others factors can operate to distinguish performance at the intermediate rates.

Fifth, clinical and laboratory measures of motor features were inversely related at a significant level, indicating that anomalous motor behavior is associated with reduced synchronization accuracy ($r = -0.53$, $p = < 0.005$). Hence, the second hypothesis – that clinical measures of motor abnormality would be associated with evidence of lower laboratory performance in motor tasks – was also supported.

The relationship between clinical evidence of formal thought disorder, as defined in this report, and laboratory measures was also analyzed. Synchronization at 80 beats/min, the rate showing the greatest spread among groups, was correlated highly with formal thought disorder ($r = 0.50$, $p < 0.005$). The relationship between formal thought disorder and synchronization at other rates was also calculated and indicates generally the same relationship – namely, that formal thought disorder was related to poorer synchronization. Hence, the third hypothesis – that performance on the laboratory task is associated with degree of formal thought disorder – was also supported. The relationship is negative and significant.

The MSTTR and synchronization accuracy were correlated at a significant level ($r = 0.35$, $p < 0.05$), indicating that reduced accuracy on the motor task is associated with evidence of language impairment.

The major finding of this study is that measures of synchronization with auditory stimuli appear to distinguish the performance of schizophrenics and controls. Because schizophrenic performance overlaps with that of controls at some rates and diverges markedly at others, neither low motivation, the effect of general psychosis, difficulty of the procedure, motor dexterity, drug effects, nor tapping speed ability satisfactorily account for the observed differences. The plausibility of these explanations depends fundamentally on their ability to operate consistently across the experimental procedures. Failing that, other explanations must be considered.

These results are, however, consistent with predictions based on the hypothesis that schizophrenics are less able than controls to take advantage of the redundancy (in the information-processing sense of the term) of the auditory stimuli in order to synchronize tapping efficiently and accurately, a process similar to that required to automate any skilled motor activity [61, 62]. The ability to be aware of and make use of the redundancy or predictability of the clicks has the effect of decreasing the need to attend to estimating click occurrence and selecting and coordinating the tapping response. Prior work summarized by Maher [63] has suggested that a disturbance in attentional focusing operates to impair the production of comprehensible speech in schizophrenics. In the synchronization procedure, a similar difficulty may disrupt performance. Specifically, we might expect that schizophrenics fail to adapt their attentional processes to the redundancies intrinsic to the task and hence exhibit relatively inefficient tapping and inaccurate synchronization. Indeed, schizophrenic performance, like that of controls, is aided by the redundancy of the stimuli, but to a significantly lesser degree.

Much work in experimental psychology has also shown that the performance of motor responses depends critically upon the operation of attentional processes [64–66]. Particular importance has been attached to the effects of attention on the timing of sequential movements [67]. Moreover, in view of the work of Sternberg et al. [68], who demonstrated a connection between language and motor control in an investigation of speech and typewriting, and Barlett's observations about the connections between language, thought, and motor movement, and their elaboration by Posner [69] into a sophisticated model pointing to the processes of attention involved in the sequencing and shifting of motor acts and thoughts, the results of the present investigation, which demonstrate a strong association between motor and language disorder that clinically have certain similarities (e. g., repetition in speech and movement) in schizophrenia, can reasonably be considered within an attentional deficit frame of reference. Yet other views may be appropriate as well and a skeptical attitude toward this as well as other explanatory models is warranted until it is better supported. Nevertheless, the possible relationship between such features and cortical and subcortical atrophy, which could be understood in the framework of an attention deficit should be explored.

Manschreck et al. [70] replicated and extended the motor synchrony study with a computer-based measuring technique. The results indicate a relationship between deficient motor synchrony and the presence of negative symptoms of schizophrenia, such as blunted affect, emotional withdrawal, and refusal to speak. Additional work is needed to understand the nature of motor synchrony, but it appears that deficient performance in this task is related to disturbances in thinking and clinical motor abnormality in schizophrenic disorders.

Abnormal Involuntary Movements (Tardive Dyskinesia)

It is now appropriate to turn attention to developments in our understanding of abnormal involuntary movements (AIMs) and, in particular, tardive dyskinesia. A varying percentage of schizophrenic and other patients who have received neuroleptic treatment exhibit a syndrome of involuntary choreoathetoid movements affecting principally the oral-buccal-lingual and facial areas and occasionally extending to the trunk and limbs [71]. Orofacial and lingual dyskinesias are the most characteristic and best recognized features of tardive dyskinesia. The source of such movements is thought to be striatal dopaminergic hyperfunction that appears to arise as a response to neuroleptic blockade of dopamine receptors. The mechanism behind the dopaminergic hyperfunction is hypothesized to be dopamine receptor supersensitivity. A corollary to this hypothesis is that dopamine receptors may be increased in the brains of patients with AIMs.

There are dissenting views on many of the commonly accepted notions about abnormal involuntary movements in schizophrenia, especially the contribution of the disease process, the clinical state of the patient, and the pathogenesis of the movements. Some of these views have a starting point in the observation that it is still not known why certain schizophrenic patients show abnormal involuntary movements during prolonged neuroleptic treatment, while others do not. There is some indication that patients with AIMs have not had longer or more intensive drug treatment than those without such movements [72]. Hence, it is possible that one or more factors inherent in the patients (rather than the treatment) predispose them to the occurrence of abnormal involuntary movements. Among such factors, *age* is the only characteristic consistently implicated. But there may be others [73].

For example, certain nonschizophrenic patients with characteristics of dementia (chronic deteriorating course and intellectual impairment) and other forms of brain disorder have been shown to exhibit involuntary movements in the absence of a history of exposure to neuroleptics. In a recent study [31], prominent orofacial dyskinesias were detected in older schizophrenic patients who had not been exposed to neuroleptic drugs. These observations appear similar to ones made by Kraepelin, Bleuler and others before drugs were available, and have increased interest in learning whether such movements may be manifestations of both disease and aging processes, independent of drug treatment. And it has called into reconsideration the prevalent view that neuroleptics cause these movements.

Studies by Waddington et al. [72] and others [73] have demonstrated several related and important findings which suggest that, among other things, schizophrenic patients with AIMs may have structural brain disturbances. Compared to those without AIMs, schizophrenic patients with AIMs show evidence of (a) intellectual impairment, (b) ventricular enlargement, and (c) association with features of the defect state or type II schizophrenia [74], often called negative symptoms – mutism prominent among them. Animal studies and postmortem studies suggest that receptor characteristics in patients with and without AIMs do not differ consistently. Wong et al.'s [75] recent PET study that showed elevated D_2 dopamine receptors in the caudate nucleus of drug-naive schizophrenics has suggested that increased receptors may be a biochemical abnormality intrinsic to schizophrenia.

It would be far fetched to suggest that all AIMs result from the disease and/or aging, rather than from the influence of neuroleptic treatment. Nevertheless, the contributions of nondrug related spontaneous involuntary movements and disease process to tardive dyskinesia have probably been underestimated. There is the possibility that neuroleptic drugs interact, possibly synergistically, with these predisposing processes in the evolution of AIMS. Hence the occurrence of AIMS in younger patients would appear to be associated with increased probability of deterioration to the defect state of schizophrenia (type II).

The disturbing prevalence of tardive dyskinesia and its association to cognitive impairment raise an important question: What is the relationship between tardive dyskinesia (AIMs) and intrinsic abnormal voluntary motor disturbances (AVMs) in schizophrenics? There are, of course, two general hypotheses that could be put forward. The first is that the two kinds of motor anomaly are independent, resulting from at least two different processes or sets of processes. The second, that they are related, assumes a common process (or set of processes) underlying their occurrence. Currently, there is no clear-cut data to help us choose between these alternatives.

Nevertheless, the latter hypothesis, that AVMs and AIMs are related, with AVMs preceding AIMs, appears plausible for several reasons. First, patients with AVMs and those with AIMs show similar problems in intellectual functioning and thought production, (i.e. the so-called defect features), and they differ largely in age and prevalence. Second, the principle of parsimony favors a single process explanation, particularly when we know so little about the underlying pathophysiology.

Several predictions might follow from this hypothesis: (1) The severity of AVMs may be a factor influencing the occurrence of AIMs (i.e. younger schizophrenics with more severe AVMs may be at higher risk for AIMs than patients with absent or lower frequencies of AVMs). (2) The occurrence of AIMs may portend a more severe course. A corollary would be that the presence of AIMs would be associated with deficits of a similar kind to those occurring in patients with AVMs but distinguished by greater severity. In line with Crow's [74] Type II proposal, the underlying or predominant abnormality in patients with persistent AIMs may be a structural deficit; in AVMs, this abnormality may be biochemical, as in the type I schizophrenia subtype.

(3) If there is, however, increased abnormality/severity in schizophrenic patients with AIMs, the cognitive performance of these patients may show qualitative (i. e. different kinds) as well as quantitative (i.e. worse) differences from those occu rring in patients with AVMs.

Preliminary Findings from an Investigation of the Relationship of AIMs and AVMs in Schizophrenic Patients

We have recently studied the clinical psychopathology, cognitive features, and neurological characteristics of a group of chronic schizophrenic outpatients (mean age 40 ± 9.5 years), who were evaluated for the presence of AIMs (dyskinesia) and AVMs (abnormalities of voluntary motor response) [76]. There were no group differences in the Beck depression scores, nor in other features of psychosis, such as delusional thinking, perceptual disturbance, and bizarre or unusual behavior. Similarly, no group differences emerged for family history of schizophrenia, abnormal EEG findings, routine CT scan abnormalities, or length of hospitalization.

The findings also showed that: (1) there were no differences in age, education, duration of antipsychotic treatment, cumulative lifetime or current dose of antipsychotic drugs between patients with and without AIMs (n = 11 and n = 10, respectively); (2) patients with AIMs had significantly greater evidence of AVMs; (3) formal thought disorder categories of poverty of information (t = 4.72, p < 0.001, two-tailed) and understandability (t = 3.93, p < 0.001, two-tailed) were also present to a greater degree in the dyskinetic grouped; (4) negative features (based on the Scale for the Assessment of Negative Symptoms (SANS) were significantly more characteristic of the group with AIMS. The greatest differences in individual features were blunting (t = 3.79, p < 0.001, two-tailed), alogia (t = 3.65, p < 0.002, two-tailed) and apathy (t = 2.40, p < 0.03, two-tailed). BPRS blunted affect ratings also parallel these differences (t = -2.53, p = 0.02).

Laboratory and Cognitive Measures

The data showed similar disturbances in the two groups for recognition memory using a signal detection paradigm, motor synchronization with an auditory stimulus, and overall recall performance in a contextual constraint task. Certain tests indicated greater deficiency in the dyskinetic group. For example, minimental state scores suggested greater difficulty in this group for simple recall. Shipley-Hartford vocabulary scores indicated that premorbid ability in patients with dyskinesia was significantly lower than those without (t = 2.25, p = 0.04, two-tailed). History of minor neurologic disturbance among dyskinetic patients was more common, bordering on significant.

Perhaps the most striking finding in the battery was the observation that AIMS patients did not prime as effectively in a lexical decision task (a measure of semantic association network activation and inhibition). On the other hand, the other patients did prime (p < 0.04). This difference is a critical one because it indicates a relative failure in cognitive performance that cannot be explained as a consequence or confound of the impaired motor activity of the dyskinesia group. It may therefore point to a more complete understanding of the associational influences operating in both motor and language production. And it may represent a means for further exploration of the nature of underlying brain disturbance in different schizophrenic groups. We have found recently [77], for example, that thought-disordered schizophrenics have priming abilities superior to nonthought-disordered schizophrenics, affective and normal controls.

These results are consistent with the hypothesis that dyskinesia (AIMs) and intrinsic schizophrenic motor abnormalities (AVMs) are related. Patients with AIMS were more likely to have greater evidence of other abnormal movements, more profound disturbances in negative or defect features, and test scores consistent with premorbid intellectual impairment. While this does not point to a specific underlying pathogenetic mechanism, it discloses the presence of a range of greater disturbances in the dyskinetic group in this group and is therefore consistent with the hypothetical relationship between AVMs and AIMs in schizophrenics. Although the results are suggestive, we are unable to conclude whether these differences represent simply more severe or different dysfunctions of schizophrenic patients.

Comment

The study of motor abnormalities must progress substantially to make a significant contribution to the neurology of schizophrenia. A critical step toward that goal will be to overcome the indirect nature of measurement of neurologic (central) abnormality through the study of behavioral (peripheral) features. Classic neurology successfully dealt with this limitation through the study of neuropathology. Investigators of schizophrenia may be able, through the use of imaging technologies, to relate behavior to central nervous system structure and/or physiology [78]. A related critical step not to be overlooked is the establishment of better, quantifiable, reliable, experimentally useful, ideally laboratory based techniques for investigation. Advances of both sorts should enrich the prospects for a mature neurology of schizophrenia.

Conclusions

The clinical and experimental literature of psychopathology of motor behavior and schizophrenia is sketchy at best. Nevertheless, important observations have been made that suggest avenues for further investigation: (1) Motor abnormalities intrinsic to schizophrenic disorder occur more frequently than generally believed. (2) Antipsychotic medications produce many motor effects, but they tend to reduce voluntary motor anomalies intrinsic to schizophrenic disorder and may not modify the occurrence of certain spontaneous involuntary disordered movements, at least among chronic cases. (3) Motor disturbances, as currently understood, are not pathognomonic for schizophrenic disorder. (4) Schizophrenic motor disturbances are associated with formal thought disorder, certain neurological signs, and affective blunting. (5) The exact relationship of motor features to prognosis is unclear. It appears, however, that the more severe the profile of motor disturbance, the more grave the illness. Observations of developmental motor difficulty in high-risk children also suggest that motor abnormalities detectable at an early age and prior to the onset of illness may portend a more severe and serious outcome. (6) Studies attempting to examine the motor and language deficits with laboratory techniques indicate an association between the two dimensions of behavior in schizophrenic disorder. They suggest parallel breakdowns in the capacity to utilize redundancy in behavior. The source of such breakdown, which can be conceptualized cognitively (attention) or neurologically (brain damage), remains a focus for research. (7) Data suggest that the abnormal involuntary movements are associated not only with drug treatment but also with the aging and disease processes. (8) Any satisfactory account of schizophrenic deficit must provide an explanation for all forms of motor disturbance.

References

1   Kleist, K.: Untersuchungen zur Kenntnis der psychomotorischen Bewegungsstörungen bei Geisteskranken (Klinkhart, Leipzig 1908).
2   Kraepelin, E.: Dementia praecox (Livingstone, Edinburgh 1919).
3   Manschreck, T.C.; Maher, B.A.; Rucklos, M.E.; Vereen, D.E.: Disturbed voluntary motor activity in schizophrenic disorders. Psychol. Med. *12:* 73 (1982).
4   Marsden, C.; Tarsy, D.; Baldessarini, R.: Spontaneous and drug-induced movement disorders in psychotic patients; in Benson, Blumer, Psychiatric aspects of neurological disease (Grune & Stratton, New York 1975).

5 Bleuler, E. (originally published 1911): Dementia praecox or the group of schizophrenias (International Universities Press, New York 1950).

6 Fish, F.: Clinical psychopathology (Wright, Bristol 1967).

7 Mailloux, N.W.; Newberger, M.: The word curves of psychotic individuals. J. abnorm. soc. Psychol. *36:* 110 (1941).

8 Wulfeck, W.: Motor function in the mentally disordered. Psychol. Rec. *4:* 271 (1941).

9 Jackson, J. (originally published, 1894): In Selected writings of James Hughlings Jackson, vol. 2 (Basic Books, New York 1958).

10 Arieti, S.: Primitive habits and perceptual alterations. Archs Neurol. Psychol. *53:* 378 (1945).

11 Jelliffe, S.: The mental pictures in schizophrenia and in epidemic encephalitis. Res. Publ. Ass. nerv. ment. Dis. *5:* 204 (1928).

12 Orton, S.T.: Some neurologic concepts applied to catatonia. Archs Neurol. Psychiat. *23:* 114 (1930).

13 Jaspers, K.: General psychopathology (University of Chicago Press, Chicago 1963).

14 Slater, E.; Roth, M.: Clinical psychiatry (Baillière, London 1969).

15 Freeman, T.: Psychopathology of the psychoses (International Universities Press, New York 1969).

16 Manschreck, T.C.: Psychopathology of motor behavior in schizophrenia. Prog. exp. Pers. Res. *12:* 53 (1983).

17 Kahlbaum, K. (originally published, 1874): Catatonia (Johns Hopkins Press, Baltimore 1973).

18 Regenstein, Q., Alpert, J.; Reich, P.: Sudden catatonic stupor with disastrous outcome. J. Am. med. Ass. *238:* 618 (1977).

19 Morrison, J.R.: Catatonia. Retarded and excited types. Archs gen. Psychiat. *28:* 39 (1973).

20 Andrews, E.: Catatonic behavior: recognition, differential diagnosis, and management; in Manschreck, Psychiatric medicine update: Massachusetts General Hospital reviews for physicians (Elsevier/North-Holland, New York 1981).

21 Gelenberg, A.: The catatonic syndrome. Lancet *ii:* 1339 (1976).

22 Mahendra, B.: Where have all the catatonics gone? Psychol. Med. *11:* 669 (1981).

23 Marsden, C.D.: Motor disorders in schizophrenia. Psychol. Med. *12:* 13 (1982).

24 Guggenheim, F.; Babigian, H.: Diagnostic consistency in catatonic schizophrenia. Schizophrenia Bull. *11:* 103 (1974).

25 Jones, M.; Hunter, R.: Abnormal movements in patients with chronic psychiatric illness; in Crane, Gardner, USPHS Publ. 1936 (1968).

26 King, H.E.: Psychomotor correlates of behavior disorder; in Kietzman, Sutton, Zubin, Experimental approaches to psychopathology (Academic Press, New York 1976).

27 Mettler, F.A.; Crandell, A.: Neurologic disorders in psychiatric institutions. J. nerv. ment. Dis. *128:* 148 (1959).

28 Allison, R.: Perseveration as a sign of diffuse and focal brain damage. Br. med. J. *I:* 1027–1032; *II:* 1095–1101 (1966).

29 Freeman, T.; Gathercole, C.: Perseveration: the clinical symptom in chronic schizophrenia. Br. J. Psychiat. *112:* 27 (1966).

30 Stengel, E.: A clinical and psychological study of echo reactions. J. ment. Sci. *93:* 598 (1947).

31 Owens, D.G.C.; Johnstone, E.C.; Frith, C.D.: Spontaneous involuntary disorders of movement. Archs gen. Psychiat. *39:* 452 (1982).

32   Feighner, J.; Robins, E.; Guze, S.; Woodruff, R.A.; Winokur, G.; Munoz, R.: Diagnostic criteria for use in psychiatric research. Archs gen. Psychiat. 26: 57 (1972).
33   Schneider, K.: Clinical psychopathology (Grune & Stratton, New York 1959).
34   Mellor, C.S.: First-rank symptoms of schizophrenia. Br. J. Psychiat. 117: 15 (1970).
35   Carpenter, W.T., Jr.; Strauss, J.S.; Muleh, S.: Are there pathognomonic symptoms in schizophrenia? An empiric investigation of Kurt Schneider's first-rank symptoms. Archs gen. Psychiat. 28: 847 (1973).
36   Pope, H.G.; Lipinski, J.F.: Manic-depressive disorders and schizophrenia. Archs gen. Psychiat. 35: 1 (1978).
37   Chapman, J.: The early symptoms of schizophrenia. Br. J. Psychiat. 112: 225 (1966).
38   Jones, I.N.: Observations on schizophrenic stereotypies. Compreh. Psychiat. 6: 323 (1965).
39   Yarden, P.E.; Discipio, W.J.: Abnormal movements and prognosis in schizophrenia. Am. J. Psychiat. 128: 317 (1971).
40   McGhie, A.: Pathology of attention (Penguin, Baltimore 1969).
41   Tucker, G.; Silberfarb, P.: Neurologic dysfunction in schizophrenia; in Akiskal, Webb, Psychiatric diagnosis (Spectrum, New York 1978).
42   Fish, B.: Biological antecedents of psychosis in children; in Freedman, Biology of the major psychoses (Raven, New York 1975).
43   Robins, L.: Deviant children grow up (Williams & Wilkins, Baltimore 1966).
44   O'Neal, P.; Robins, L.: Childhood patterns predictive of adult schizophrenia. Am. J. Psychiat. 115: 385 (1958).
45   Watt, N.: Childhood and adolescent routes to schizophrenia; in Ricks, Thomas, Roff, Life history research in psychopathology, vol. 3 (University of Minnesota Press, Minneapolis 1974).
46   Ricks, D.; Nameche, G.: Symbiosis, sacrifice, and schizophrenia. Ment. Hyg. 50: 541 (1966).
47   Ricks, D.; Berry, J.: Family and symptom patterns that precede schizophrenia; in Roff, Ricks, Life history research in psychopathology, vol. 1 (University of Minnesota Press, Minneapolis 1970).
48   Marcus, J.: Cerebral functioning in offspring of schizophrenics. Int. J. ment. Hlth 3: 57 (1974).
49   Mednick, S.A.; Mural, M.; Schulsinger, G.; Mednick, B.: Perinatal conditions and infant development in children with schizophrenic parents. Soc. Biol. 18: 108 (1971).
50   Hanson, D.; Gottesman, I.; Heston, L.: Some possible childhood indicators of adult schizophrenia inferred from children of schizophrenics. Br. J. Psychiat. 129: 142 (1976).
51   Erlenmeyer-Kimling, L.; Cornblatt, B.; Friedman, D.; Marcuse, Y.; Rutschmann, J.; Simmens, S.; Devi, S.: Neurological, electrophysiological, and attentional deviations in children at risk for schizophrenia; in Henn, Nasrallah, Schizophrenia as a brain disease (Oxford University Press, New York 1982).
52   Manschreck, T.C.; Maher, B.A.; Ader, D.N.: Formal thought disorder, the type-token ratio, and disturbed voluntary motor movement in schizophrenia. Br. J. Psychiat. 139: 7 (1981).
53   Manschreck, T.C.; Maher, B.A.; Rucklos, M.E.; Vereen, D.R.; Ader, D.N.: Deficient motor synchrony in schizophrenia. J. abnorm. Psychol. 90: 321 (1981).
54   Breil, M.S.: Graphologische Untersuchungen über die Psychomotorik in den Handschriften Schizophrener. Mschr. Psychiat. Neurol. 125: 193 (1953).

55   Kneutgen, J.: Experimentelle Analyse einer Wahrnehmungsstörung bei Schizophrenie: Desynchronisation von Handbewegungen mit einer gleichformigen akutischen Frequenz. Fortschr. Neurol. Psychiat. *44:* 182 (1976).

56   Cromwell, R.L.: Stimulus redundancy in schizophrenia. J. nerv. ment. Dis. *146:* 360 (1968).

57   Maher, B.A.; Manschreck, T.C.; Rucklos, M.: Contextual constraint and the recall of verbal material in schizophrenia: The effect of thought disorder. Br. J. Psychiat. *137:* 69 (1980).

58   Manschreck, T.C.; Maher, B.A.; Rucklos, M.E.; White, M.: The predictability of thought-disordered speech in schizophrenic patients. Br. J. Psychiat. *134:* 595 (1979).

59   Spitzer, R.; Endicott, J.; Robins, E.: Research diagnostic criteria for a selected group of functional disorders (RDC) (Biometrics Research, New York 1975).

60   Lundin, R.: An objective psychology of music (Ronald Press, New York 1967).

61   Posner, M.; Keele, S.W.: Attention demands of movements; in Proceedings of the 17th Congress of Applied Psychology (Zeitlinger, Amsterdam 1969).

62   Schmidt, R.A.: Anticipation and timing in human motor performance. Psychol. Bull. *70:* 631 (1968).

63   Maher, B.A.: The language of schizophrenia: a review and interpretation. Br. J. Psychiat. *120:* 3 (1972).

64   Ells, J.G.: Analysis of attentional and temporal aspects of movement control. J. exp. Psychol. *99:* 10 (1973).

65   Rosenbaum, D.A.: Human movement initiation: Specification of arm, direction, and extent. J. exp. Psychol. *109:* 444 (1980).

66   Stelmach, G.F.: Information processing in motor control and learning (Academic Press, New York 1978).

67   Rosenbaum, D.A.; Pastashnik, D.: A mental clock setting process revealed by reaction time: in Stelmach, Requin, Tutorials in motor behavior (North Holland, Amsterdam 1980).

68   Sternberg, S.; Monsell, S.; Knoll, T.L.; Wright, C.E.: The latency and duration of rapid movement sequences: Comparisons of speech and typewriting: in Stelmach, Information processing in motor control and learning (Academic Press, New York 1978).

69   Posner, M.I.: Orienting of attention. Qu. J. exp. Psychol. *32:* 3 (1980).

70   Manschreck, T.C.; Maher, B.A., Waller, N.G.; Ames, D.M.: Latham, C.A.: Deficient motor synchrony in schizophrenic disorders: Clinical correlates. Biol. Psychiat. *20:* 990 (1986).

71   Tarsy, D.; Baldessarini, R.: Tardive dyskinesia. A. Rev. Med. *35:* 605 (1984).

72   Waddington, J.L.; Youssef, H.A.; Molloy, A.G.; O'Boyle, K.M.; Pugh, M.: Association of intellectual impairment, negative symptoms, and aging with tardive dyskinesia: clinical and animal studies. J. clin. Psychiat. *46:* 29 (1985).

73   Baldessarini, R.J.; Cole, O.J.; Davis, J.M.; Gardos, G.; Preskorn, S.H. et al.: Tardive dyskinesia: summary of a task force report of the American Psychiatric Association. Am J. Psychiat. *137:* 1163 (1980).

74   Crow, T.J.: Molecular pathology of schizophrenia: More than one disease process? Br. med. J. *280:* 66 (1980).

75   Wong, D.F.; Wagner, H.N.; Tune, L.E.; Dannals, R.F.; Pearlson, G.D.; Links, J.M. et al.: Positron emission tomography reveals elevated D_2 dopamine receptors in drug-naive schizophrenics. Science *234:* 1558 (1987).

76   Manschreck, T.C., Keuthen, N.; Schneyer, M.L.; Collins, P.; Laughery, J.: Abnormal in-
      voluntary movements and schizophrenic psychopathology. (submitted).
77   Manschreck, T.C.; Maher, B.; Milavetz, J.; Ames, D.; Weisstein, C.; Schneyer, M.L.:
      Semantic priming in thought-disordered schizophrenic patients. Schizophrenia Res. *1:*
      61–66 (1988).
78   Guenther, W.; Breitling, D.; Banquet, J.P.; Marcie, P.; Rondot, P.: EEG mapping of left
      hemisphere dysfunction during motor performance in schizophrenia. Biol. Psychiat. *21:*
      249 (1986).

Theo C. Manschreck, MD, Laboratory of Clinical and Experimental Psychopathology,
Massachusetts General Hospital, Harvard Medical School, Boston, MA 02114 (USA)

Therapeutic Aspects of Movement

Kirkcaldy B (ed): Normalities and Abnormalities in Human Movement.
Med Sport Sci. Basel, Karger, 1989, vol 29, pp 128–146

Movement Quality Changes in
Psychopathological Disorders

Harald G. Wallbott

Department of Psychology, University of Giessen, FRG

Quantitative and Qualitative Aspects of Human Movement

'Abnormal psychomotor behavior is often the most visible and most dramatic first sign of psychopathology' [Nathan et al., 1969, p. 3]. Given this argument, of the central role of movement characteristics in psychiatric descriptions of some psychopathological states, consistent with postulations in the earliest psychiatric textbooks of, for instance, Bleuler or Kraepelin (see below), an attempt will be made in this chapter to present some evidence from the literature. Futhermore, a comprehensive discussion is offered of methodological and technical aspects of studying movement behavior.

Reduced to its *physical* aspects, each visible movement can be described by the way an object or an (idealized) point characterizing this object, travels in the three spatial dimensions between the onset and end of the respective movement, thus adding time as the forth dimension. Hence, each movement can be considered as consisting of coordinate changes in the three spatial dimensions in time. Within a movement the *spatial* changes may be large or small, *velocity* and *acceleration* may change during the course of the movement, and with respect to the dimension of *time* movements may be short or long. This can be considered as the most basic level of movement description.

On another level, movements can be described with respect to *form* or to *function*. Systems to describe movements with respect to its form were predominantly developed in nonpsychological disciplines, one example being dance notation systems [cf. Laban, 1975, and the chapter by Lyons and Pope, this vol.] attempting to describe movements in as much detail as possible, allowing another person to precisely replicate the described movements. A similar approach involving exhaustive description of movement behavior was presented by Birdwhistell [1970]. He attempted to describe the form of movements by providing categories of possible movements for each part of the human body able to move independent of other bodily parts.

Systems attempting to classify human movements with respect to its function require category systems defining different functional units. Ekman and Friesen [1969, 1972], for instance, attempted to code movement behavior with only five large functional categories (with subclassifications introduced for each of these categories): *illustrators*, which are movements tightly linked to speech, i.e. accentuating, punctuating, stressing what is said (mainly hand and head movements); *adaptors* or *manipulators*, which reflect basic needs or arousal of an organism (for instance 'nervous' hand movements); *emblems*, which are movements with precise meaning [see Ekman, 1975] which can be readily translated into speech (like for example, the 'victory' gesture or the 'shrug'); *regulators*, which are movements that help to structure and organize interactional conduct, such as movements used to initiate speaking turns, and finally *affect displays*, which are movements indicative of emotions and states of the organism, particularly evident in human facial movements.

Another influential functional classification of movements (though restricted to hand movements) was developed by Freedman and co-workers [Freedman et al., 1973; Freedman, 1977]. In their functional classification they stress the different relations of movements to speech by basically distinguishing between 'object-focussed' movements (tightly related to speech encoding) and 'body-focused' movements (with less close relationships to speech). Both major categories are further differentiated into sets of subcategories.

A third level to describe movements besides the physical level, and the 'form or function' level is the level of *impression*, describing not the physical characteristics of movements but perceived qualities of movements. Movement quality, i.e. the way in which human movements are executed with respect to the dimensions of time and space is mentioned as an important diagnostic aspect of psychopathological disorders both in the old German 'expression psychology' [Asendorpf and Wallbott, 1982; Wallbott, 1982a] and in the psychiatric literature. Literature in psychiatry, movement analysis, dance studies, and the above-mentioned 'expression psychology' reveals a large number of verbal descriptions of movement quality. Efron [1941] described gestures in terms of movement quality by using such labels. Later, Birdwhistell [1970] had included 'motion qualifiers' in his kinesics' system for the description of human movement behavior: 'intensity', 'range', and 'velocity'.

The poetic, impressionistic descriptions of movement such as 'angular' or 'jerky' also appear very important in lay psychology. People judge other person's gait as being clumsy or jerky, their handshakes as weak or strong, or their gestural behavior as being fidgety or tense. Often, attributions about personality traits or states are based on such judgements.

Especially in the psychiatric literature such descriptions are treated as if they were objective and valid descriptions of movement behavior. For example, a psychiatrist describing a patient's movement behavior as being jerky, angular, and abrupt, or the behavior of the same patient after successful therapeutic attempts as showing rounded and even movements does not describe the patient's movement quality objectively, but instead relies on his subjective impressions of movement behavior. In order to appreciate the potential diagnostic value of such descriptions, it has to be demonstrated that: (a) Such verbal labels can be used reliably by independent observers of movement behavior. (b) Such descriptions are systematically related to objectively measurable movement characteristics like their velocity, acceleration, or circumference. (c) Descriptions and related objective movement characteristics are valid diagnostic indicators for the classification of different diagnostic groups (cf. schizophrenics vs. depressives) or for the evaluation of a patient's improvement during the course of therapy.

A model which allows a clear distinction between objective movement characteristics and subjective impressions and descriptions, the 'lens model', was developed by Brunswik [1956]. Scherer [1978] has extended Brunswik's original model to specifically describe *impression formation* processes [see also Cline, 1964]. This model states that impression formation may be divided into three processes. The first one relates a criterion (for instance, a psychopathological state) to distal cues, defined as objectively measurable behavioral cues and predicted to be associated with the criterion. This externalization process is followed by the actual perception process: objective distal cues are perceived by an observer and subjectively represented as proximal cues. Finally, these proximal cues are combined in the attribution or impression formation process to result in an inference or attribution of the sender's state.

When all components are measured separately, it is possible to specify relations within the model via correlation coefficients, which provide answers to questions of veridicality (relation between criterion and attribution), accuracy of perception of distal cues (relations between distal and proximal cues), criterion validity of distal cues as indicators of the criterion, and finally the impact of proximal cues on the attribution. As far as the topic of this chapter is concerned, psychopathological state can be considered as the criterion, objectively measured movement parameters represent the distal cues (as for instance velocity, circumference, etc.), subjective movement judgements (rounded, angular, expansive, etc.) represent proximal cues, and the attribution of psychopathological state or a 'diagnosis', the attribution part of the model.

Within the framework of this model the following questions can be asked: (a) Is the psychopathological state associated with objective characteristics of movement quality? (b) How are subjective movement descriptions, i.e., proximal cues, used by observers and how are these related to distal, objective movement cues? (c) To what extent do distal and proximal cues contribute to a diagnosis, i.e., are movement cues useful in judging psychopathological state? (d) Finally, what is the relation between the criterion 'psychopathological state' and the corresponding attributions? Can psychopathological state be judged accurately using movement cues and if so, which cues are important in these judgements?

Later we will give an example of a study which tried to follow this general paradigm. Before doing so we will selectively review some results from psychiatry and psychology concerning relationships between movement characteristics and psychopathology.

Studies on Movement Quality in Psychiatry

From the beginning of modern psychiatry, movement behavior constituted one important aspect of symptomatology [cf. Kraepelin, 1883; Bleuler, 1949; Kretschmer, 1921]. Some diagnostic categories are centrally based on motor behavior, especially catatonia. Psychiatrists like Oseretzky [1931] have even devised special test batteries to diagnose psychopathological disturbances on the basis of motor behavior [cf. Vandenberg's chapter].

Modern nonverbal behavior research has followed that tradition and shown that there appear to be systematic relationships between movement aspects and psychiatric diagnoses on the one hand and improvement ratings after therapy on the other. The work of Ekman and Friesen [1972, 1974], Freedman and Hoffman [1967], Freedman [1977], and of Ulrich [1977, 1979], who applied Freedman's coding technique, indicates that movement behavior, especially gestural behavior, is a useful indicator of psychopathological state. Depressive patients in particular seem to be characterized by fewer illustrative (speech-accompanying) gestures compared to schizophrenics or normal controls. Furthermore, degree of improvement in patients is associated with more illustrative hand movements and less body-focussed, manipulative hand movements (such as scratching oneself). Though these studies yielded important insight into the function of nonverbal behavior in psychopathology, they concentrated mainly on quantitative aspects of the occurrence of certain classes of hand movements (like illustrators or manipulators), but neglected the qualitative aspects of movement.

As previously mentioned, psychiatric descriptions focus on such qualitative characteristics. We will give just a few examples: Wolff [1951] characterizes movements of schizophrenics as being 'disturbed, abrupt, halted, stilted', occasionally 'staccato-like', sometimes with 'over-emphasis'. Ruesch and Kees [1956, p. 166] describe 'angular, jerky, uncoordinated movements carried out with uneven acceleration and deceleration and at either too slow or too fast a tempo...' of schizophrenic patients. Arieti [1959] as well as Spiegel [1959] have observed 'stereotyped motions' and 'impulsive gestures' of schizophrenics. Millon [1969, p. 499] describes schizophrenics' movement behavior in a similar fashion, being characterized by 'motor retardation', 'stereotyped repetitive acts, bizarre gestures, rapid, irregular and jerking motions'. In the same way, Burgoon and Saine [1978] emphasize the 'jerky and uncoordinated movements' of schizophrenics.

For depressive patients similar descriptions of movement abnormalities may be found. Here usually the aspect of 'motoric retardation' is of central interest [Davidson and Neale, 1974; Frese and Schöfthaler-Rühl, 1976; Fischer-Cornelssen and Abt, 1980], that is, a general reduction in movement activity or in movement velocity. Arieti [1959] mentions 'psychomotor retardation... actions decrease in number... and even those which are carried out are very slow' [p. 426]. In the extreme case of depressive stupor, movements are 'definitely inhibited or suppressed' [p. 437]. Spiegel [1959] stresses the general reduction of gesticulation in depression, and Coleman and Broen [1972] consider 'decreased motor activity' as a central symptom in depression.

Of course, these qualitative descriptions of movement behavior are by no means unambiguous. The observed differences between schizophrenics and depressives for instance, do not seem to be as clear as one might expect. Miller [1975, p. 246], for example, states that 'however, depressives are not more retarded than schizophrenics'. Similarly, Weitbrecht [1960] stresses that movement abnormalities are an important symptom of psychopathology, but that similar movement characteristics may be observed across all types of psychiatric disorders. When studying the relation of 16 symptoms of 'abnormal psychomotor behavior' to psychiatric diagnoses, Nathan et al. [1969] only found positive correlations with the general label 'psychosis', but not with specific diagnostic classifications. Lang and Buss [1965, p. 100] concluded from similar results: 'There is ample evidence that severity of psychopathology and psychological deficit are positively related, ... some theorists hold that this is the only meaningful relationship between deficit and diagnosis, and they argue that specific consideration of schizophrenia is superfluous.' Miller [1975] further found that motor abnormalities of depressives cannot be considered as being typical for this diagnosis, but only for general psychopathology.

Thus we may conclude that movement characteristics are more indicative of the *degree* of psychopathology, and less of the *type* of psychopathology.

None of these issues has been studied extensively in an objective fashion. Movement quality descriptions in the psychiatric literature usually relate proximal cues (the descriptions) directly to a criterion (diagnosis or state) without considering the mediating distal cues, i.e. objective movement characteristics. Because of this neglect, the issue of which distal cues (if any) impressionistic movement judgements are based on, remains unresolved. Brengelmann [1960, p. 98] stated with respect to this problem: 'It may be argued that the emphasis on judgement of expressive qualities of movement has distracted attention from the actual measurement of movement. Although judgement of movement has opened up extremely fruitful avenues of research, emphasis on movement *per se* should be revived.'

Johansson [1973] was one of the few who studied the relations between distal and proximal movement cues by demonstrating that subjective judgements of different types of human locomotion (like running, jumping, walking) are strongly associated with distinctive patterns of objective movement parameters. Waxer [1974, 1976] was almost the only one to show that the attribution of depression was both valid in terms of a criterion 'depression' (established via MMPI data) and reliably associated with distal nonverbal behavior cues such as reduced duration of eye contact, head bent forward, or reduced gestural behavior. These results indicate that at least in principle, observers are able to accurately infer psychopathological state and that they use nonverbal cues and especially movement cues in this process. Thus, it should be possible to specify exactly which movement characteristics result in inferences of movements being for instance, 'stiff, angular, rounded, etc.'.

Studies on Movement Quality in Expression Psychology

Another source of information on movement quality aspects as a diagnostic tool is provided by a successor of modern nonverbal communication research, the German 'expression psychology' [for a detailed overview, see Asendorpf and Wallbott, 1982; Asendorpf, 1982; Wallbott, 1982a; Helfrich and Wallbott, 1986]. Though expression psychology was less concerned with the expression of psychopathological states in movement behavior, but rather dealt with the expression of personality or 'character', some of the results are relevant for our topic. Expression psychology presents a lot of studies trying to describe differences in movement quality between pycnics (with a 'cyclothymic character', relating this personality type to depression – similar to Sheldon's [Sheldon and Stevens, 1942] endomorphic temperament) and leptosomics (with a 'schizothymic character' related to schizophrenia – similar to Sheldon's ectomorphic temperament), such character types drawn mostly from the work of Kretschmer [1967].

Movement quality of pycnics in these studies is usually described as being 'soft, rounded, fluent, without inhibitions' [Enke, 1930], or as being 'natural, fluent, uninhibited' [Geiger, 1935; Strehle, 1960]. Takala [1972] characterized pycnic persons by rather slow and more regular movements. Schizothymics on the other hand present 'precise, angular, rigid, and hasty' movements [Enke, 1930], or 'faster, more expansive, and angular' movements [Geiger, 1935; Strehle, 1960].

Such results were obtained especially when studying gait and gestures of subjects with different personality types. An overview of this line of research is given in Wallbott [1982a, p. 28], where the differences in movement quality between pycnics (the personality type which according to Kretschmer is related to depression) and leptosomics (related to schizophrenia) were summarized as follows: pycnics – more rounded, gentle, harmonic, elegant, and graceful movements; leptosomics – more restricted, stiff, angular, cramped, and tense movements. Some of these results resemble the differences reported between movements of schizophrenics and depressives discussed above.

As in the psychiatric studies on movement quality mentioned, the major problem of these results is that the differences found are often anecdotal or rather subjective interpretations and labels of movement behavior. As mentioned from time to time in this chapter, movement descriptions like 'stiff' or 'angular' are not objective data, but *interpretations* of movement characteristics. Given research and observations, movement quality seems to be an important diagnostic cue. But in order to more fully understand the nature of objective characteristics of movements leading to impressions of for instance, 'angular' movements, the physical parameters and objective measurement techniques required for analyzing movement behavior have to be better understood. In the next section we will attempt to selectively review some of these parameters and measurement techniques [for a more elaborated overview, see Wallbott, 1980, 1982b].

Measurement Techniques for the Study of Movement Behavior

When surveying techniques for measuring movement behavior, a broad distinction can be made between 'direct' measurement approaches and 'indirect' approaches [Wallbott, 1980].

Direct measurement techniques include all those techniques involving direct attachment of a monitoring device to the moving subject under observation. Thus, direct techniques include electromyographic measurements of muscle potentials with surface or needle electrodes attached to the relevant muscles as well as such devices as tremometers [Enke, 1930], force plates [Paul, 1975], goniometers [Bishop and Harrison, 1977], or infrared movement detectors [Sainsbury and Wood, 1977]. Usually such techniques are very exact in measuring movement, but on the other hand rather obtrusive to subjects, because electrodes etc. have to be carried around. This obtrusiveness renders such techniques problematic in certain situations and they may be difficult to administer to certain patient groups. Furthermore, the equipment required is extremely elaborate and thus rather costly both in terms of instrumentation and time needed for analysis.

In contrast to such direct approaches, 'indirect' approaches include all assessment methods, where movement is 'measured' (to be understood in the broadest sense) by an observing device, this device being a human observer, judging movement characteristics, or a recording device allowing storage of movement behavior for further analysis. We [Wallbott, 1980, 1982b] have proposed structuring such indirect techniques on a dimension ranging from global, subjective descriptions of movements to fully automated computerized systems for movement analysis, which at least conceptually, do not require a human observer. We will briefly review some of these techniques, providing one or two references for each application [for details, see Wallbott, 1980].

Coding/description techniques (inference by a human observer as an integral part of the measurement procedure):

(a) Phenomenal descriptions, global judgements of movement behavior without explicit, defined categories, as frequently used in psychiatry and expression psychology (see above) [cf. Jacobson, 1936; Klages, 1964].

(b) Phenomenal descriptions with explicit, but not fully operationalized categories [Kietz, 1956; Kiener, 1962].

(c) Category approaches or functional classifications using explicit, operationalized categories (coding systems for gestural behavior etc. used in nonverbal communication research, for instance Ekman and Friesen's [1969] functional categories of illustrators, manipulators, emblems, etc., or Freedman et al.'s [1973] distinction between object-focussed and body-focussed movements).

(d) Transcriptions of movement behavior or notation systems, attempting to describe human movement behavior in as much detail as possible, permitting replication of movements by other persons, the origin often being dance notation systems or approaches that use transcription techniques from general linguistics [Laban, 1975; Preston-Dunlap, 1969; Birdwhistell, 1970].

(e) Transcription and notation systems that make use of technical facilities to obtain more reliable descriptions and classifications, for instance Frey and Pool's [1976] system which allows insertion of cross-hairs into a video-recording, facilitating more exact coding of movements with respect to the three spatial dimensions.

Methods for the analysis of recorded/stored movement behavior, using 'subjective' interpretations by description or categorization:

(a) Special photographic and motion picture techniques like interrupted light photography, stroboscopy, or serial photographs (nowadays in most applications bypassed by modern video technology, the 'ancestors' being Marey [1894] and Muybridge [1901]; more modern applications reported by Jones and Narva [1955] and Waterland [1968]).

(b) Sketches or drawings from film or video tape [Efron, 1941; Hopper and Kane, 1968].

(c) Usage of film projectors with facilities like slow motion, stop motion, frame-by-frame projection, etc. (now somewhat outdated by modern video equipment facilities, though resolution of 16 mm film seems to be better than resolution of standard (VHS) video equipment [Wallbott, 1982c; for applications, compare Condon, 1970; and Galle, 1975].

Methods for the analysis of recorded/stored movement behavior, with 'objective' interpretation by computing physical parameters:

(a) Time-way graphs obtained by frame-by-frame projection following defined points of moving body parts in time 'by hand', subjects often wearing markers attached to their bodies to allow better identification of defined points on the recording (again a somewhat outdated technique, examples being Efron [1941] and Kietz [1956]).

(b) Time-way graphs obtained by the same manual technique (frame-by-frame projection and marking of points by hand), but processed into physical parameters of movements, sometimes semiautomatic processing of coordinate data [Fischer, 1911; Smith, 1975; Chapman and Borchardt, 1977; Wallbott, 1985].

(c) Time-way graphs obtained by merely automatic devices. These techniques require light-emitting diodes or other marks, whose signals can be traced by automatic cameras or detectors, attached to the moving body. Thus, this method is rather obtrusive [Mitchelson, 1975; Hoenkamp, 1978].

(d) Pattern recognition and automatic feature detection (advanced techniques not yet used in psychological or psychiatric research on human movement behavior [see Bond, 1975]).

In the following section of this chapter we will report about a study employing both objective quantitative analysis of movement quality (coordinate measurements) and subjective judgements of movement quality for comparing movement behavior of depressive patients prior to and after successful therapy.

An Illustrative Study

Movement quality may be assessed for different types of movement, e.g., gestures or gait. In the study to be reported here it was decided to focus attention on hand illustrators [Ekman and Friesen, 1972], i.e., hand movements accompanying, illustrating, and accentuating the verbal content of utterances. This choice was motivated both by issues concerning psychological theory as well as technical reasons. It has been shown that the frequency of use of hand illustrators is related to psychopathological state. Thus, it seemed interesting to determine whether quality of movement would show similar effects. Technically, illustrators are, besides gait, '... the most frequent, regularly occurring, quantifiable... bits of overt behavior available for objective study' [Freedman, 1977, p. 112]. Illustrators are large in spatial extension and usually of some temporal duration. Because of this extension in time and space, which renders them highly suitable for quantitative measurement as well as for judgement studies (easy visibility), hand illustrators were selected for analysis.

This study was based on video-records of psychiatric patients' behavior [details are reported in Wallbott, 1982b, 1984, 1985]. Patients were filmed shortly after their arrival at the hospital (= admission, i.e. in a 'sick' condition) and shortly before they were about to leave the hospital when they were judged as much improved by psychiatrists (= discharge). For the recording a semistandardized interview was conducted of about 6–10 min duration. Camera angle and placement of the camera were similar for all recordings [for details see Ekman and Friesen, 1968]. The results are derived from a sample of 20 patients diagnosed as being primarily depressed.

Two trained coders experienced in the coding of nonverbal behavior, especially in Ekman and Friesen's system for the coding of hand-movement behavior [Friesen et al., 1979], localized each illustrative hand movement independently of one another in the total corpus of 40 interviews. From this sample of about 250 illustrators, 60 items were selected from the admission interviews and 60 from the discharge interviews. The sample contained only illustrators executed primarily in the horizontal (left-right) and the vertical (up-down), but not in the frontal (to and away from the camera) spatial dimension, because the system used for quantitative analysis of movement (see below) offered analysis of only two spatial dimensions. The 120 scenes with illustrators thus selected were edited onto a new video-tape in random order across patients and across the criterion admission-discharge. Thus, this study was not concerned with patients' diagnoses, nor with changes of individual patients' behavior during therapy. The aim was to compare illustrators before and after successful therapy, in order to study movements, not patients.

The methods available for the analysis of human movement behavior have already been described. For the measurement of distal movement parameters, coordinate measurements seem to be most appropriate. For the present study, a system was devised allowing for coordinate measurements directly from existing video recordings. A 'video pointer' (FOR-A Co., Japan) connected to a video-recorder inserts an arrow into the video picture; this arrow can be moved to any point of the picture via a joystick. The system enables registration of the two spatial coordinates (horizontal and vertical) of the arrow's point. These coordinates were digitized using an A/D converter and stored on a PDP 11/35 mini-computer.

The system is operated by a coder. When a movement has been localized, the video-recorder is placed into frame-by-frame mode at the onset of the movement. Then the arrow is moved to a particular point, coordinates of which are stored (here the proximal knuckle of the middle finger); storage of coordinates follows by depressing a switch. The recorder is subsequently moved to the next frame and so forth, until the movement is terminated. Agreement between independent coders using the system was higher than 90% [for details, see Wallbott, 1982b].

The data were stored in the computer as pairs of consecutive coordinate readings, one number representing the position relative to the horizontal (left-right) dimension, the other relative to the vertical (up-down) dimension. Using mathematical, pythagorean operations these XY data can be transferred into temporal, spatial, and spatiotemporal parameters [Wallbott, 1980]. The following well-established parameters in kinesiology research [cf. Hinson, 1977] were used: (1) *temporal* parameters: duration of movement; (2) *spatial* parameters: total waylength, total and mean circumference, maximum reach [Efron, 1941], and (3) *spatiotemporal* parameters: mean and maximum velocity, mean and maximum acceleration, maximum deceleration, mean jerk (changes in acceleration), maximum acceleration increase, maximum deceleration increase, and the standard deviations of velocity, acceleration, and jerk as parameters for the 'steadiness' of movements.

All parameters were computed from video-frame to video-frame, i.e. between each two consecutive coordinate pairs both for the X- and Y-dimension separately and for the actual way the hands moved from frame to frame, which can be computed from X- and Y-coordinates by using: $r(i) = SQRT (Delta\, x(i) ** 2) + (Delta\, y(i) ** 2)$, (x(i) and y(i) being coordinate values at time i; r(i) being the way between sample points i and i-1). Where necessary these data were then averaged for each movement (cf. mean velocity; for details see Wallbott, [1982b]).

Proximal cues of movement quality were studied in terms of movement descriptor adjectives like 'angular, jerky, or fast' as used in psychiatry and expression psychology. Natural language provides a nearly infinite number of these terms, thus a sample had to be selected. From a pool of 107 terms collected from the nonverbal behavior literature [cf. Efron, 1941], from psychiatry and expression psychology [Wallbott, 1982a], from dance- and movement-notation literature [cf. Hutchinson, 1977], and from dictionaries and thesauri, 18 were eventually selected as being representative items to describe gestural behavior. The terms finally selected in order of appropriate judgements were the following: lively, tense, clumsy, vehement, uncontrolled, fidgety, expansive, energetic, jerky, hurried, brisk, unrestrained, jittery, intense, abrupt, fast, smooth, angular. Using the resulting 18 scales, a questionnaire was devised which allowed judgements of the 120 illustrator scenes on 9-point scales (0 = not at all ...; 8 = very much ...); 20 judges watched the stimulus tape and rated the 120 scenes on the 18 scales of movement quality. In line with the design suggested by the lens model as a final step, attributions whether a certain scene was judged as stemming from an admission or a discharge interview were obtained. The judges were asked to decide for each of the 120 scenes whether they thought it was taken at admission or prior to discharge.

One issue under study was whether observers would agree on the use of movement description terms like 'angular' or 'jerky' or whether such judgements would be used randomly across observers. Results [for details, see Wallbott, 1985] indicate that the judgements were not purely random. Some scales like 'lively, expansive, fast, vehement' reached substantial reliability. It is interesting that those scales which describe 'simple' physical characteristics of movements such as 'expansive' (extension in space), 'fast' (velocity), 'vehement' (energy?) were used with more agreement. Scales which indicate more complex, 'Gestalt' aspects of movement quality for example, 'jittery, clumsy, uncontrolled, or angular' are used with rather low agreement by judges. Unfortunately, the latter terms are the ones that are most frequently used in psychiatry and expression psychology!

Correlations between judgement and objective movement data provide evidence for the notion that judges inferred movement quality, using perceived physical characteristics of movements. Movements judged as more 'smooth' for example, are characterized distally by large circumference, long waylength, high mean velocity, but no abrupt changes in velocity or acceleration (standard deviations of velocity and acceleration). Thus, 'smooth' movements seem to be large in terms of space and exhibit a high but even velocity. 'Hasty' movements in turn are characterized mainly by high mean velocity, and high mean acceleration. Finally, to name another example, 'expansive' movements show high correlations with all circumference and waylength parameters, indicating that these objective movement characteristics strongly determine judgements of the respective proximal cue ('expansive').

Having shown that proximal judgements of movement quality can be used in a reliable fashion and that such judgements are valid with respect to objective distal movement characteristics, we now have to test whether both distal and proximal movement measurement really reflect changes in patients' state during the course of therapy as frequently hypothesized in psychiatric literature. When testing admission-discharge differences for the distal coordinate parameters, it is rather striking that none of the coordinate parameters studied differentiates between admission and discharge. This failure to find significant differences indicates that movement quality as measured here, at least for this particular sample of patients, does not have any relation to admission-discharge differences in patient state.

In contrast, when looking at admission-discharge differences in the proximal judgements, some highly significant differences emerge [see Wallbott, 1985]. Movements at discharge were judged as being significantly more 'hurried, fast, lively, brisk, fidgety, uncontrolled, unrestrained, and jerky' compared to movements at admission. Thus, in terms of proximal judgements, movements at discharge are more 'hasty', but there are virtually no differences for intensity, space, and more especially fluency-course between admission and discharge, though hypotheses from psychiatry and expression psychology would have predicted just that.

Comparing attributions to distal parameters it was found that those movements judged to be from discharge interviews rather than from admission, display a larger mean circumference and larger maximum reach; they are of higher mean and maximum velocity, as well as of higher acceleration, higher jerk, and higher standard deviations for the respective parameters. Thus, the attributions are related to the distal cues, while the criterion is not!

It has been demonstrated that the criterion was only related to judgements of movements at discharge, being faster, more hurried, etc., compared to movements at admission. Interestingly, the correlations between proximal judgements and attributions point into exactly the opposite direction. Movements judged as taken from discharge compared to movements judged as being from admission are perceived as more intense, more expansive, and markedly less angular, smoother, less jittery, tense, and clumsy. Thus, movements *believed* to be from discharge differ significantly from movements believed to be from admission in intensity, space, and fluency-course, while there are no correlations with 'hastiness', which in turn was the only aspect substantially associated with the criterion!

The judgements of admission-discharge resulted in invalid attributions compared to the criterion, even though both distal and proximal cues were strongly related to the attributions. The only cues associated with the criterion were the hastiness judgements, but these were apparently not used in the attributions. Observers obviously did not consider that only hastiness was relevant, but instead based their attributions on the irrelevant proximal cues of fluency-course, space, and intensity and on the associated distal cues, particularly circumference and waylength parameters. Thus, the judgmental strategy employed is plausible and very similar to movement descriptions in psychiatry and expression psychology, but it is quite misleading in terms of the objective admission-discharge criterion.

Movements after successful therapy are *not* of larger circumference or longer waylength or higher velocity, nor are they smoother, less angular, more intense or more expansive. But observers seem to have based their attributions on just that inaccurate assumption. They judged movements as being from a discharge interview, when they in fact were of higher circumference or when they were judged as being less angular. This policy resulted in totally invalid attributions since none of the cues used bears a relationship to the criterion. This account of an invalid judgement policy demonstrates the usefulness of a lens model design in studying clinical judgement. Observers were not 'wildly guessing'. On the contrary, they used a very logical and stringent judgement policy, but one which was based on the wrong premises.

With respect to the clinical framework of the study it has been shown that admission-discharge attributions based on gestural behavior were totally invalid. Together with the results on reliability and validity of proximal cues this implies that the attributions were based on invalid distal and proximal cues. The approach presented here not only allowed detection of the usage of invalid cues, i.e., an answer to the question, why the attributions were not accurate, but also determination of those cues used, leading to invalid attributions.

This approach allows detailed analysis of the processes of cue utilization and cue misutilization and to identify cues relevant and irrelevant for correct and (more importantly) for incorrect attributions. In an applied sense, this enables judges to focus attention for instance in clinical practice, on cues which are valid in terms of a criterion and to correct attributions based on invalid cues.

Final Remarks

We have attempted in this chapter to provide an overview of movement quality aspects as indicators of psychopathological state as well as on measurement methods for describing movements. Though in psychiatric literature descriptions of movement quality as indicators of psychopathological state are by no means rare, empirical studies testing the assumption of movements as valid indicators of psychopathological state are scarce. In fact, in our own study, evidence that movement parameters were systematically related to patients' improvement was lacking except the well-known fact that movements of depressive patients were executed faster after successful therapy. Observers on the other hand thought that movements that were less jittery, less clumsy, but more expansive to name just a few examples, stemmed from a discharge interview. Though observers' impressions were not valid in this study, they resemble remarkably descriptions in the literature on movement characteristics of psychiatric patients.

This is not to say that psychiatrists or psychologists describing movement characteristics as indicators of pathological states or clinical improvement are wrong or use cues as inaccurately as our judges did. Our study was restricted to one type of movement behavior (hand illustrators), only some (though central) distal and proximal cues, and to a rather small sample of depressive patients.

But generally it has to be kept in mind that most clinical diagnoses are based on inferences and that the proximal cues leading to such inferences should, as far as possible, be validated by studying objective distal cues. This is not only true for cues of movement quality as described here, but for all diagnoses based on inferences from patients' behavior.

Of course most of the techniques for movement analysis described in this chapter are rather costly, both in terms of time and equipment, and thus are probably unsuitable for clinical practice. But some of the methods reported were developed and widely used for rehabilitation and sports' research [see for instance Chapman and Borchardt, 1977; for an overview, see Wallbott, 1982b]. Though these techniques for movement analysis have been rather successfully used in these applied areas, applications in the area of clinical psychology or psychiatry are rare. It was our aim here to emphasize the pressing need for more basic research on the relationships between movement behavior and clinical states, especially as a safeguard for not basing diagnoses on (sometimes wrong or inaccurate) subjective impressions! The techniques to study movement behavior are available, so why should we not use them?

References

Arieti, S.: Manic-depressive psychosis; in Arieti, American handbook of psychiatry, pp. 439–454 (Basic Books, New York 1959).

Asendorpf, J.: Contributions of the German 'expression psychology' to nonverbal behavior research. 2. Facial expression. J. nonverb. Behav. 6: 199–219 (1982).

Asendorpf, J.; Wallbott, H.G.: Contributions of the German 'expression psychology' to nonverbal behavior research. 1. Theories and concepts. J. nonverb. Behav. 6: 135–147 (1982).

Birdwhistell, R.L.: Kinesics and context (University of Pennsylvania Press, Philadelphia 1970).

Bishop, E.; Harrison, A.: A demonstration of modular units in motor programming? J. hum. Movem. Stud. 3: 99–109 (1977).

Bleuler, E.: Lehrbuch der Psychiatrie; 8th ed. (Springer, Berlin 1949).

Bond, C.P.: Television image analysis. Res. Film *8:* 439–443 (1975).

Brengelmann, H.: Expressive movements and abnormal behavior; in Eysenck, Handbook of abnormal psychology, pp. 62–107 (Pitman Medical, London 1960).

Brunswik, E.: Perception and the representative design of psychological experiments (University of California Press, Berkeley 1956).

Burgoon, J.K.; Saine, T.: The unspoken dialogue (Houghton-Mifflin, Boston 1978).

Chapman, A.E., Borchardt, W.: Biomechanical factors underlying the dislocate on still rings. J. hum. Movem. Stud. *3:* 221–231 (1977).

Cline, V.B.: Interpersonal perception; in Maher, Progress in experimental personality research, vol. 1, pp. 221–284 (Academic Press, New York 1964).

Coleman, J.C.; Broen, W.E.: Abnormal psychology and modern life (Scott, Foresman, Glenview 1972).

Condon, W.S.: Method of micro-analysis of sound films of behavior. Behav. Res. Meth. Instrument. *2:* 51–54 (1970).

Davidson, G.C., Neale, J.M.: Abnormal psychology: An experimental-clinical approach (Wiley, New York 1974).

Efron, D.: Gesture and environment (King's Crown, New York 1941); new edition: Gesture, race, and culture (Mouton, The Hague 1972).

Ekman, P.: Movements with precise meaning. J. Commun. *26:* 14–26 (1975).

Ekman, P.; Friesen, W.V.: Nonverbal behavior in psychotherapy research; in Shlien, Research in psychotherapy, vol. III, pp. 179–216 (APA, Washington 1968).

Ekman, P.; Friesen, W.V.: The repertoire of nonverbal behavior: Categories, origins, usage, and coding. Semiotica *1:* 49–98 (1969).

Ekman, P.; Friesen, W.V.: Hand movements. J. Commun. *22:* 353–374 (1972).

Ekman, P.; Friesen, W.V.: Nonverbal behavior and psychopathology; in Friedman, Katz, The psychology of depression: Contemporary theory and research, pp. 203–232 (Winston, Washington 1974).

Enke, W.: Die Psychomotorik der Konstitutionstypen. Z. angew. Psychol. *36:* 238–287 (1930).

Fischer, O.: Methodik der speziellen Bewegungslehre; in Tigerstedt, Handbuch der physiologischen Methodik, vol. 3, pp. 120–316 (Hirzel, Leipzig 1911).

Fischer-Cornelssen, K.A.; Abt, K.: Videotape recording in psychiatry and psychopharmacology. Acta psychiat. scand. *61:* 228–238 (1980).

Freedman, N.: Hands, words, and mind: On the structuralization of body movements during discourse and the capacity for verbal representation; in Freedman, Grand, Communicative structures and psychic structures, pp. 109–132 (Plenum, New York 1977).

Freedman, N.; Blass, T.; Rifkin, A.; Quitkin, F.: Body movements and the verbal encoding of aggressive affect. J. Pers. soc. Psychol. *26:* 72–85 (1973).

Freedman, N.; Hoffman, S.P.: Kinetic behavior in altered clinical states: Approaches to objective analysis of motor behavior during clinical interviews. Percept. Mot. Skills *24:* 527–539 (1967).

Frese, M.; Schöfthaler-Rühl, R.: Kognitive Ansätze in der Depressionsforschung; in Hoffmann, Depressives Verhalten, pp. 58–97 (Müller, Salzburg 1976).

Frey, S.; Pool, J.: A new approach to the analysis of visible behavior (Research Reports from the Department of Psychology, Bern 1976).

Friesen, W.V.; Ekman, P.; Wallbott, H.G.: Measuring hand movements. J. nonverb. Behav. *1:* 97–112 (1979).

Galle, H.K.: Die Methodik der herkömmlichen Filmauswertung. Res. Film *8:* 409–420 (1975).

Geiger, E.: Zur Psychomotorik der Konstitutionstypen bei industriellen Hämmerarbeiten (Triltsch, Würzburg 1935).

Helfrich, H.; Wallbott, H.G.: Contributions of the German 'expression psychology' to nonverbal behavior research. 4. The voice. J. nonverb. Behav. *10:* 187–204 (1986).

Hinson, M.M.: Kinesiology (Brown, Dubuque 1977).

Hoenkamp, E.C.M.: Perceptual cues that determine the labelling of human gait. J. hum. Movem. Stud. *4:* 59–69 (1978).

Hopper, B.J.; Kane, J.E.: Analysis of film – The segmentation method. Biomechanics *1:* 42–44 (1968).

Hutchinson, A.: Labanotation (Theatre Art Books, New York 1977).

Jacobson, W.: Charaktertypische Ausdrucksbewegungen. Z. pädag. Psychol. *37:* 307–317 (1936).

Johansson, G.: Visual perception of biological motion and its analysis. Percept. Psychophys. *14:* 201–211 (1973).

Jones, F.P.; Narva, M.: Interrupted light photography to record the effect of changes in the poise of the head upon patterns of movement and posture in man. J. Psychol. *40:* 125–131 (1955).

Kiener, F.: Hand, Gebärde und Charakter (Reinhardt, München 1962).

Kietz, G.: Der Ausdrucksgehalt des menschlichen Ganges (Barth, Leipzig 1956).

Kiritz, S.A.: Hand movement and clinical ratings at admission and discharge for hospitalized psychiatric patients; diss. San Francisco Medical Center (1973).

Klages, L.: Grundlegung der Wissenschaft vom Ausdruck (Bouvier, Bonn 1964).

Kraepelin, E.: Psychiatrie (Barth, Leipzig 1883).

Kretschmer, E.: Körperbau und Charakter (Springer, Berlin 1921/25th ed. 1967).

Laban, R.: Principles of dance and movement notation; 2nd ed. (MacDonald & Evans, London 1975).

Lang, P.J.; Buss, A.H.: Psychological deficit in schizophrenia. 2. Interference and activation. J. abnorm. Psychol. *70:* 77–106 (1965).

Marey, E.J.: Le movement (Masson, Paris 1894).

Miller, W.R.: Psychological deficit in depression. Psychol. Bull. *82:* 238–260 (1975).

Millon, T.: Modern psychopathology (Saunders, Philadelphia 1969).

Mitchelson, D.L.: Recording movement without photography; in Grieve, Miller, Mitchelson, Paul, Smith, Techniques for the analysis of human movement, pp. 33–65 (Lepus, London 1975).

Muybridge, E.: The human figure in motion (Dover, New York 1901).

Nathan, P.E.; Zare, N.; Simpson, H.F.; Andberg, M.M.: A systems analytic model of diagnosis. 1. The diagnostic validity of abnormal psychomotor behavior. J. clin. Psychol. *25:* 3–9 (1969).

Oseretzky, N.I.: Psychomotorik: Methoden zur Untersuchung der Motorik. Z. angew. Psychol. *57:* suppl. (1931).

Paul, J.P.: Instruments for force measurement; in Grieve, Miller, Mitchelson, Paul, Smith, Techniques for the analysis of human movement, pp. 150–171 (Lepus, London 1975).

Preston-Dunlap, V.: A notation system for recording observable motion. Int. J. Man-Machine Stud. *1:* 361–386 (1969).

Ruesch, J.; Kees, W.: Nonverbal communication (University of California Press, Berkeley 1956 re-issued 1972).

Sainsbury, P.; Wood, E.: Measuring gesture: Its cultural and clinical correlates. Psychol. Med. *7:* 63–72 (1977).

Scherer, K.R.: Personality inference from voice quality: The loud voice of extraversion. Eur. J. soc. Psychol. *8:* 467–487 (1978).

Sheldon, W.H.; Stevens, S.S.: Varieties of human temperament (Harper, New York 1942).

Smith, A.J.: Photographic analysis of movement; in Grieve, Miller, Mitchelson, Paul, Smith, Techniques for the analysis of human movement, pp. 3–29 (Lepus, London 1975).

Spiegel, R.: Specific problems of communication in psychiatric conditions; in Arieti, American handbook of psychiatry, pp. 909–949 (Basic Books, New York 1959).

Strehle, H.: Mienen, Gesten und Gebärden (Reinhardt, München 1960).

Takala, M.: The communication of personal styles. Reports from the Department of Psychology, University of Jyväskylä (1972).

Ulrich, G.: Videoanalytische Methoden zur Erfassung averbaler Verhaltensparameter bei depressiven Patienten. Pharmakopsychologie *10:* 176–182 (1977).

Ulrich, G.: Über den Zusammenhang videoanalytisch gewonnener Masse des non-verbalen Verhaltens mit selbst eingeschätzter Befindlichkeit. Schweiz. Arch. Neurol. Neurochir. Psychiat. *125:* 349–359 (1979).

Wallbott, H.G.: The measurement of human expression; in von Raffler-Engel, Aspects of nonverbal communication, pp. 203–228 (Swets & Zeitlinger, Lisse 1980).

Wallbott, H.G.: Contributions of the German 'expression psychology' to nonverbal behavior research. 3. Gait, gestures, and body movement. J. nonverb. Behav. *7:* 20–32 (1982a).

Wallbott, H.G.: Bewegungsstil und Bewegungsqualität (Beltz, Weinheim 1982b).

Wallbott, H.G.: Audiovisual recording procedures, equipment, and troubleshooting; in Scherer, Ekman, Handbook of methods in nonverbal behavior research, pp. 542–579 (Cambridge University Press, Cambridge 1982c).

Wallbott, H.G.: Ein halbautomatisches Verfahren zur Ermittlung quantitativer Bewegungsparameter aufgrund von Videoaufzeichnungen. Motorik *7:* 110–117 (1984).

Wallbott, H.G.: Hand movement quality: A neglected aspect of nonverbal behavior in clinical judgment and person perception. J. clin. Psychol. *41:* 345–359 (1985).

Waterland, J.C.: Integration of movement. Biomechanics *1:* 178–187 (1968).

Waxer, P.H.: Nonverbal cues for depression. J. abnorm. Psychol. *83:* 319–322 (1974).

Waxer, P.H.: Nonverbal cues for depth of depression: set vs. no set. J. Consult. clin. Psychol. 44: 493 (1976).

Weitbrecht, H.J.: Depressive und manische endogene Psychosen; in Gruhle, *Psychiatrie der Gegenwart*, vol. 2, pp. 73–118 (Springer, Berlin 1960).

Wolff, C.: *The hand in psychological diagnosis* (Methuen, London 1951).

Harald G. Wallbott, PhD, Justus-Liebig-Universität, Fachbereich 06 Psychologie, Otto-Behaghel-Strasse 10, D–6300 Giessen (FRG)

Kirkcaldy B (ed): Normalities and Abnormalities in Human Movement.
Med Sport Sci. Basel, Karger, 1989, vol 29, pp 147–165

Constructs in Motion
Some Reflections on the Potential Interplay between the Notions
of Rudolf Laban and George Kelly in the Context of Therapy

S. Lyons, M. Pope

Department of Educational Studies, University of Surrey, Guildford, UK

Movement in Focus

The use of 'expressive arts' in therapy has, as Feder and Feder [1981]
pointed out, roots which can be traced back as far as the ancient Egyptian
priest-physicians and in the writings of Greek philosophers such as Plato and
Aristotle. However, their role has had a chequered history and concepts such
as mind-body dualism and the debasement of the body so prevalent in the
Victorian era have impeded full exploitation of their potential. Modern
psychotherapists acknowledge the importance of 'nonverbal behaviour' but
in practice most psychotherapy '... is still verbal and rests on the implicit
assumption that the psyche resides in the head and must be approached in
the language of the head – words' [Feder and Feder 1981, p. 12].

The theoretical bases underpinning current practice are extensive –
'medical' models, behaviourist, psychoanalytic, existentialist and humanistic
viewpoints to name but some. Verbalization plays an important role in all of
these. Differences in theoretical orientation will lead to differing degrees of
acceptance of the potential role of nonverbal formulations and differences as
to the aim of therapeutic practice.

Our own perspective is that therapeutic practice should help the client to
identify his/her problem. Such an approach necessitates a phenomenological
stance and it is recognized that verbal comment is one medium whereby the
client's understanding of the problem and personal meanings can be
revealed. However, there are occasions when both therapist and client can be
'lost for words' and at such times a systematic analysis of movement could
play an important part in the process.

In focussing on movement analysis we do not seek to deny the importance of other therapeutic practices. In this chapter we wish to highlight the work of two theorists – Laban and Kelly – whose philosophical positions may offer a source of inspiration for therapists who wish to encourage their clients to demonstrate their agency through movement. This seems appropriate since both men were interested in the possibility of people making sense of the world in a personally meaningful way, both valued experience and understanding above an 'accumulative fragmentalism' view of knowledge and recognized the potential limitation of verbal articulation in communication.

We would wish to make a case for the significance of movement observation and analysis in the therapeutic process. We do so from our joint interest in the works of Rudolf Laban and George Kelly [see also Pope and Keen, 1982, and Lyons, 1985]. It is our contention that sensitivity to movement adds to therapeutic practice. We feel unhappy that in some therapist/ client relationships emphasis on 'verbalization' obscures potentially rich sources of information.

One of Barfoot's [1980, p. 182] characters in *Gaining Ground* observed that: 'Look, you can sit here and tell me every moment of your life that you can remember, and you can analyse all of it and tell me what each moment meant to you; but there is no way I'll understand exactly because I haven't had the experiences. And I can't explain to you how it is with me because you haven't experienced what I have. We can get a sense of each other, but we can't know each other, we can't really understand. That's not so terrible; it seems to me that the sense we have of each other is quite a lovely thing. There's no need to force it into being something else.'

The sense we have of each other has a lot to do with nonverbal interaction. We are concerned that verbal discourse has numbed our sensitivity to such interaction and has assumed preeminence as a communication medium particularly in 'academic' circles.

Best [1978, p. 146] has observed that: 'those who argue for the supremacy of movement as a means of communication put themselves in an ironically self-defeating position, since it is worth noting that they themselves employ the resources of *verbal* language in order to propound their case'.

This presents a double-bind for those keen to advance the importance of movement as a medium of communication. Benthall [1975, p. 11] has noted that: 'since our society uses words as its primary means of control, all repressed groups will tend to find their most effective and confident expression through the body's wider resources rather than within the enclosure of language'.

The legacy of body/mind distinctions has been the less serious treatment of claims for movement which has conspired to marginalize movement as a physical domain. In many cases the subordination of movement has also reflected personal experiences of movement education of an aversive nature. We believe that reflection on our own movement experiences can help unlock our *epistemological projects* which in themselves are founded upon our *ontological assumptions*.

By 1925, Ferenczi was beginning to question traditional models of therapy which employed passive association techniques which took as a starting point any psychic superficies present and then worked back to preconscious cachexes of unconscious material. He called this 'analysis from above' and contrasted it with his own approach, the 'active' method, which he characterized as 'analysis from below' [Lowen, 1971, p. 11 ff.]. Within the active method can be seen the framework of a somatic approach to therapy. Lowen [1971, p. 15] has summarized the implications thus: 'The character of the individual as it is manifested in his typical pattern of behaviour is also portrayed on the somatic level by the form and movement of the body. The sum total of the muscular tensions seen as a gestalt, that is, a unity, the manner of moving and acting constitutes the "body expression" of the organism. The body expression is the somatic view of the typical emotional expression which is seen on the psychic level as "character".'

We suggest that sensitivity to movement in everyday life can enhance our understanding of our selves and others. In making the case for movement observation and analysis we are conscious of Best's [1978] exhortations about the 'slipperiness' of movement. Whilst we do not wish to make a 'wide' claim for movement as of ineluctable, universal importance, we do wish to argue that structured observation of quantitative and qualitative dimensions presents the skilled observer with information about individuals that is as significant as their verbal utterances. We recognize that *intention* and *action* are a basis for understanding movement but we do submit that the work of Laban, Lamb and others provides an insight into how a movement portrait of an individual can be constructed. In North's [1972, p. 6] terms: 'Movement, as revealed in our gestures, unconscious movements, body carriage and our working actions is always 'ourselves'. It always speaks honestly, or by its counteractions of superimposed phrases reveals that an act (conscious or unconscious) is being put on.'

In the remainder of this chapter we discuss the insights to be gained from the works of Laban and Kelly in respect of therapeutic practice. Both men brought innovative approaches to the study of human behaviour based upon their ability to observe critically. They were both practitioners: Laban worked in the worlds of dance, education and industry, whilst Kelly worked as a clinician and educator.

Our point of departure is Kelly's view of clinical assessment. He maintained that the formation of a diagnosis is not simply a matter of forming a pre-emptive construction of the individual case. Categorization does play a role in the clinician's understanding of the case but is not the end in itself. Clinical assessment is likely to be a multifaceted procedure with the ultimate aim of the development of a plan of action (treatment). Sensitivity to nonverbal behaviour is important in this process as Stefan and Linder [1985, p. 203] have indicated: 'The responsibility of the clinician is to create an atmosphere in which the individual is free to describe himself. Even if he has difficulty expressing himself in words or in actions, he must be the focus of concern and information must come from him.'

Limiting therapy to 'talking the cure' runs the risk of discarding significant information. We suggest that *structured and disciplined analysis* of movement rather than ad hoc observation can play a central rather than peripheral role in therapy. Personal construct therapists following Kelly's lead and movement analysts utilizing Laban's ideas may find it of interest to adopt an interdisciplinary approach, to consider some of the cross-currents inherent in each and perhaps generate an alternative source of inspiration for their respective projects.

Rudolf Laban

Laban was born in 1879 in Poszony, Hungary. He provided details of his life up to 1935 in his *Ein Leben für den Tanz* [translated into English by Lisa Ullman in 1975 as *A Life for Dance*] in which he characterized himself as a 'dance master' and emphasized the centrality of dance in his life. By 1928, Laban had devised and developed a system of dance notation which has subsequently been referred to as Kinetography Laban or Labanotation. Some years later, Laban acknowledged the openness of the system to 'improvement' and suggested that 'A system of notation cannot arise from the solitary endeavour of one person only' [Hutchinson, 1972, p. xv]. For Laban the ultimate aim of his notation system was to establish a literature of movement and dance. Ullman [1975, p. 184] has suggested that: 'From the earliest years of his career, Laban was convinced that dance could only gain an equal position among the other arts if it had a notation whose principles were universally applicable.'

Kinetography Laban or Labanotation provides a system for the detailed recording of movement. Hutchinson [1972, p. 11] describes the process of recording movement thus: 'The conversion of the elements of space, time, energy and the parts of the body involved into symbols which can be read and converted into movement.'

Labanotation is a comprehensive system which identifies: directional destination; motion; anatomical change; visual design; relationship; centre of weight, balance; dynamics, and rhythm pattern. In essence, Labanotation provides a written record of movement and an analysis of movement based upon a 'common language' of symbols.

In 1938, Laban came to England and spent the remaining 20 years of his life exploring his interests in human movement. Of particular significance was his study *Effort* written in collaboration with Lawrence in 1947. Their study was focused on industrial work practices but has been subsequently developed as a framework with which to analyse the qualitative aspects of movement. In the United States this form of analysis became known as Effort-Shape [Dell, 1970]. Laban and Lawrence [1974, p. 7] argued that: 'Although the practical application of the new knowledge of human effort in industry differs from that in education, art and other fields of human activity, the fundamental principles remain the same.'

An effort notation system was devised to record movement. Fundamental to this process was the assumption that: 'A person's efforts are visibly expressed in the rhythms of his bodily motion. It thus becomes necessary to study these rhythms, and to extract from them those elements which will help us to compile a systematic survey of the forms effort can take in human action' [Laban and Lawrence, 1974, p. 2].

Effort was understood by Laban to be the inner function originating movement. In Laban's terms, practically everyone has the ability to discern effort: 'We can gather the meaning of a movement and though it seems to be difficult to express it in exact words, rhythm conveys something by which we are influenced [Laban and Lawrence, 1974, p. 3]. He added that: 'Unconscious effort-reading is the explanation for our belief that we can see the thoughts and feelings shown in facial expression, in body carriage, and in the almost imperceptible expressive movements of hands, shoulders, and so on' [p. 6].

Movement was to be understood (and analysed) as outward expression of living energy within. Those who developed Effort-Shape Notation created a vocabulary with which to describe movement systematically. Variety in movement is determined by the way the mover concentrates his/her effort.

This is how Dell [1970, p. 11] describes effort: 'Effort may, at any particular moment, be concentrated in the changes of the quality of the tension, or the *flow* of movement; it may be concentrated in changing the quality of the *weight*, or the quality of *time* in the movement; or it may be concentrated in the mover's focus in *space*.'

Flow, weight, time and space are 'effort factors' and are always present in movement as quantities. There are in addition eight 'effort qualities' and they are noted by Dell [1970, p. 12] thus: 'Changes in the *flow of tension* can be either *free* or *bound*; the quality of the *weight* can become either *light* or *strong*; the quality of *time* can become either *sustained* or *sudden*; and the quality of the *spatial* focus or attention, either *indirect* or *direct*.'

We defer discussion of Laban's work here. For the moment we wish to indicate that he developed both quantitative and qualitative systems for the recording and analysis of movement. His work was of seminal importance to the development of dance and movement education in Britain. His legacy has been the provision of systems of notation which characterize the complexity of movement in a range of contexts.

Lamb [1965] has developed systematic observation of physical behaviour which distinguishes between posture and gesture. He argues that: 'We communicate through our physical behaviour before we open our mouths... yet we are little educated in physical behaviour' [p. 126ff.]. Lamb's system is extended by sensitivity to variation of movement involving shape and effort. A later work, *Body Code – The Meaning of Movement* [1979] opened up the notion of posture and gesture to a wider audience.

North [1972] has applied Laban-inspired concepts to the study of personality assessment. She argues that from a carefully compiled series of recorded movement patterns and rhythms, a movement portrait can be assembled. Comprehensive movement observation identifies use made of body, space and effort. Such observation has been used in work study, education and therapy.

Bernstein [1986] has provided a detailed account of how insights gained from Laban and Lamb have informed the emergence of movement assessment profiles particularly in the work of Kestenberger. The grounding of effort – shape in a developmental perspective, has, for Bernstein, become an invaluable tool in movement therapy.

In a tribute to Laban on the centenary of his birth, Bodmer [1979, p. 7] observed that: 'Laban was a man of such vision that it is difficult to understand the deeper implications of his work. He realised the unity of body and mind in human movement... Through this his movement observation has never been on the purely physical level but has aimed at the deepest levels of the understanding of personality.'

Foster [1960, p. 25] has suggested that Laban 'was primarily interested in people and that he developed his analysis in order to be able to discern their needs and develop their powers'.

There is much in Laban's theorizing that resonates with the approach of Kelly. We conclude our brief discussion of Laban by drawing attention to the developmental nature of his theorizing. Thornton [1971] has noted that Laban wanted each person to interpret his theories in a highly individualistic way. Skelly [1979] has added: 'I do not think that Laban ever pretended to be working within the strict parameters of a discipline or to be establishing immutable absolutes' [p. 30], and concluded that 'Laban's work will only risk stasis, the antithesis of the man, when it becomes the object of "bogus religiousity" instead of becoming an invaluable set of tools of enormous potential. Laban's work is about change, is an agent of change, and therefore must change itself' [p. 40].

George Kelly

Kelly rejected the notion of psychological theories as absolute blueprints of human nature. He offered his Personal Construct Theory as one possible way of helping make sense of human functioning. He recognized the potential of theories as tools to help understanding but saw the danger of their use as limiting cages which could stultify creative and alternative exploration. His readers were asked to consider his ideas 'as if' they may have something meaningful to offer and then to adopt or modify them in the light of further experimentation with them. It is perhaps worth noting that amongst some clinical psychologists, his work has indeed become the focus of 'bogus religiousity' rather than seen as a hypothesis to be put to the test and as a springboard for further work.

During his career as a clinical psychologist and educator, Kelly developed a psychology of personal constructs that celebrated human agency. Kelly [1969, p. 31] was quite clear in his antagonism towards a psychology which sees man as reactive rather than constructivist: 'A psychology that pins its anticipations on the repetitions of events it calls "stimuli", or on the concatenations of events it calls "reinforcements", can scarcely hope to survive as man's audacities multiply.'

For Kelly, the construction of reality is an active, creative, rational, emotional and pragmatic affair. He rejected the absolutist view of truth and contrasted his philosophical position of *constructive alternativism* with that of the dominant philosophy of *accumulative fragmentalism*: 'Constructive alternativism holds that man understands himself, his surroundings and his potentialities by devising constructions to place upon them and then testing the tentative utility of these constructions against such ad interim criteria as the successful prediction and control of events' [Kelly, 1966, p. 1].

Kelly rejected the idea of the person as an 'impotent reactor' whose behaviour is determined by environmental circumstances or genes. He preferred to portray people as active agents capable of making things happen and able to construct events; his was a self-determining model as opposed to the deterministic models which were prevalent in his lifetime. Kelly was also concerned about the nomothetic emphasis of psychometric research and the extent to which the therapist's view of the problems shaped the analysis and procedures used within the therapy. Nomothetic research does little to help the therapist deal with the individual client, and the presuppositions and theoretical framework held by the therapist may hinder progress by placing an inappropriate definition of 'the client's problem'. For Kelly, the client's definition of the problem was important and ought to be elicited. He maintained that 'if you don't know what is wrong with the patient ask him, he may tell you' [Kelly, 1955, p. 323].

Kelly's approach to the development of a person was based upon the metaphor of 'man-the-scientist'. He invited us to entertain the possibility that looking at people *as if* they were scientists might illuminate human behaviour. Person-the-scientist and scientist-the-person are both engaged in a process of observation, interpretation, prediction and control. According to Kelly, each person erects for himself a representational model of the world, and this model enables him/her to chart a course of behaviour in relation to it. The model is subject to change over time, since constructions of reality are constantly tested out and modified to allow better predictions. Thus, for Kelly, the questioning, exploring and revising in the light of predictive failure (which is symptomatic of scientific theorizing) is precisely what a person does in his or her attempts to anticipate events. Just as the scientist designs experiments around rival hypotheses, so each of us can be seen designing our daily explorations of life around rival hypotheses which form part of our system of constructs or 'world-view'. People can be seen as scientists, constantly experimenting with their definitions of existence.

People may construe their environment in an infinite number of ways, depending on their imagination and the courageousness of their experimentation. Kelly did not deny the importance of early experiences or present environmental circumstances, but he suggested that it was more important to know what and how people think about their present situation – that is, their current hypotheses/constructs – than to know what their early childhood experiences were or what environmental circumstances they now find themselves in. Rather than see people as trapped by their early experiences or present environmental constraints, Kelly suggested that individuals be encouraged to see their hypotheses or *representational models* open to refutation. These representational models are composed of a series of interrelated personal constructs or tentative hypotheses about the world. Constructs are used by a person to describe present experience, to forecast events *(theory building)*, and to assess the accuracy of previous forecasts after the events have occurred, thereby testing predictive efficiency *(theory testing)*.

Kelly's main emphasis was on the uniqueness of each person's construction of the world and on the construct system that each involves, and continues to evolve, in order to impose meanings on his or her experiences. He devised a Repertory Grid Technique to elicit constructs and explore personal construct systems. Beail [1985, p. 2] describes Kelly's approach thus: 'Kelly's original role Construct Repertory Test, from which all subsequent forms of grid derive, was designed to elicit a representative sample of personal constructs upon which an individual relies to interpret and anticipate the behaviour of significant people in their life, and to assess the way in which they relate their constructs one to another.'

Bannister and Fransella [1980, p. 65] have indicated that the original grid technique probably drew on Kelly's knowledge of mathematics in order to yield a mathematical relationship between constructs. They note however that: 'Kelly did not think methods of quantification were all there should be in the psychologists' tool-bag. Constructs can be elicited from an individual in conversation, from essays, from poetry, from journal papers.'

Kelly also employed the *self-characterization* sketch as a method that invited clients to say something about themselves. As Bannister and Fransella [1980, p. 76] point out: 'The aim is to find out how the person structures their immediate world, how they see themselves in relation to these structures and the strategies they have developed to handle their world.'

Pope [1981] has drawn attention to the problems created by an overzealous application of quantitative grid techniques. In particular, there are inherent difficulties in requiring individuals to give verbal labels in order to articulate constructs. Kelly himself pointed out that it is a mistake to equate constructs with the verbal labels used to identify them. Some individuals may find it exceedingly difficult to put into words their thoughts and feelings. We argue that grid techniques have a *limited range of convenience* and that by recognizing the developmental aspect of personal construct psychology and applying approaches which seek to make use of subjective meaning therapeutic practice can be advanced.

Just as Laban invited the refinement of his ideas, so too did Kelly avoid programmatic statements about personal construct psychology. There would be a fundamental contradiction in Kelly's work if frameworks based on constructive alternativism achieved a prescriptive and static quality. Novak [1985, p. 5] has noted that: 'Any notion of people as personal scientists needs to move beyond what Kelly wrote and to look at what he actually was doing. To stick to what Kelly wrote in 1955 would be limiting and very unKellyan.'

Movement in Personal Construct Therapy

We believe that Laban and Kelly offer, within their *philosophical* positions, a rich source of inspiration that goes beyond the structures they devised. Both men were ultimately interested in the possibilities of people making sense of the world within which they lived. Laban focused his attention on movement as a fundamental aspect of nonverbal interaction. In doing so he established an agenda for the study of movement as a unity of physical, mental and spiritual dimensions. For Kelly, the psychotherapist or teacher, in carrying out their facilitative role, would be engaged in a process whereby the client/learner could recognize his/her agency and responsibility for the models of the world he or she had created and in this way the person would not be 'a victim of biography'.

Despite the fact that Repertory Grid methods and self-characterization sketches rely on verbal formulation, Kelly [1955, p. 16] recognized that: 'A person is not necessarily articulate about the construction's he places upon his world. Some of his constructions are not symbolised by words; he can express them only in pantomime. Even the elements which are construed may have no verbal handles by which they can be manipulated and the person finds himself responding to them with speechless impulse. Thus in studying the psychology of man-the-philosopher we must take into account his sub-verbal patterns of representation and construction.'

The personal construct therapist may find considerable difficulty in facilitating the expression of these nonverbal constructions. Movement analysis may play a part in overcoming such problems. Epting [1981, p. 192] in his appraisal of personal construct psychotherapy suggested that most of the attention in experimental research in personal construct psychology has 'concentrated on the construct in its most tightened form: the verbal labels obtained from various forms of Role Construct Repertory Test'. However, Epting [1981, p. 192] argues that in therapy we may be dealing with constructs which remain at low levels of awareness and may be preverbal: 'These may be constructs which were either formed before the client had a verbal system or are new constructs that enter into the client awareness, at first, only as vague feelings and very loosely formulated understandings... an important feature of them is the way they are first noticed as body sensation... This feature points to the fact that all constructs are embodied. In construct theory there is no mind of construct dimension separate from a body of sensations. We badly need better techniques to get at these dimensions in therapy.'

We suggest that the recognition of moving as a means of construing and the potential of movement analysis may provide a vehicle for a person's reflective understanding. It may also act as a mode of communication between therapist/educator and client as an adjunct or an alternative to more traditional verbal therapies. We do not, of course, wish to characterize therapy as a solely verbal exchange. But by adopting an approach to our being-in-the-world which challenges existing therapeutic practice we seek to explore the role movement therapy has to play albeit recognizing current limitations in this field. We are concerned that the process of matching therapeutic modality with the client includes movement as an option. As Chaiklin and Schmaiss [1986, p. 20] have noted, the significance of dance as direct communication is in the 'externalisation of those inner feelings which cannot be expressed in rational speech but can only be shared in rhythmic, symbolic action'.

In the ensuing discussion we wish to note some of the extant literature on the use of movement in therapy and then to explore developments in constructive psychology. It should be noted that potential links between Kelly and Laban's notions and their interplay in therapy are at a very formative stage and the reader is invited to consider them further.

As we indicated earlier, a tradition for the inclusion of movement in therapy was already established in the 1920s. Since that time there have been a number of movement 'therapies' which have made claims for inclusion in the therapeutic process. Warren [1984] has noted that approaches to therapy can be characterized as part of a continuum which range from the mental/medical at one end to the experiential/human growth at the other. Feder and Feder [1981] have identified how dance/movement therapists have struggled for acceptance in the United States and have sought professional credibility. In some senses, the use of dance as a creative art in the therapeutic process represents an acceptable face of movement therapy. In the United States, pioneers of dance/movement therapy were Chace and Whitehouse. Both came to be involved in therapy from a background in dance. Chace was the first president of the American Dance Therapy Association in 1965. She explored the therapeutic use of dance in her work at St. Elizabeth's Hospital in Washington, D.C. Whitehouse [1986] acknowledged the impetus given to her own work by Chace in the development of her own therapeutic use of 'authentic movement'. Significantly, Whitehouse [1986, p. 63] argued that: 'In order to find out what it was that truly moved people, I needed to give up images in them and in myself of what it meant to dance... to dance surely meant the making of a product, finishing a piece of work to show. I was finding more and more that the things happening in classes allowed pieces of movement, not dances; and that it would be more directly descriptive to call what the people were doing movement until such time as they themselves wanted to make dances.'

Others involved in the development of dance therapy included Schoop, Espenak and Bartenieff [Bernstein 1986].

Schoop [1974] has argued from a autobiographical basis for the inclusion of dance in therapy. Her book *Won't You Join the Dance?* recounts her attempts to communicate with chronic schizophrenics in dance. She reports that: 'It seems to me that each body I see radiates its own nonverbal message, and that message represents the sum total of the individual's various characteristics' [p. 61]. By working on a one-to-one basis, Schoop strove to encourage new and positive feelings about the self. Her system of therapy focused on: breathing, alignment, centrality, tension and rhythm. She is concerned that 'we don't always want to listen to what the body has to report' [p. 44].

One of the problems to be faced by movement therapy has already been identified: the low status attached to 'physical' activity. Social and cultural changes have further devalued our knowledge of our selves through movement. Despite what some observers have regarded as the fetishization of the body in consumer cultures we seem to operate at a superficial level in our understanding of nonverbal interaction.

In academic circles there have been demands for those involved in movement to provide 'objective' statements about the subjective experience of movement. Personal experiences of kinaesthesia are private, inner-directed and self-referential. If movement in or as therapy is to challenge conventional wisdom then the double-bind alluded to earlier must be addressed. A growing body of literature is providing credibility for claims made for movement.

Individuals have to learn verbal and nonverbal systems of interaction. Kinesics is an attempt to address issues in nonverbal interaction. Birdwhistell [1973] suggests, for example, that body motion is a learned form of communication which is patterned within a culture and which can be broken down into an ordered system of isolable elements. Condon [1968] and others have discovered ordered and rhythmical physical elements in speech. Speakers and listeners develop a *synchrony* of movement that is finely tuned. Feder and Feder [1981, p. 163] report that Kestenberg has explored the early development of interactional behaviours. She has found that infants and mothers engage in reciprocal holding patterns from which emerges mutual trust: 'The *trustworthy* baby does not lean on the mother so heavily that she cannot breathe in comfort, nor does the *trustworthy* mother hold him in a rigid embrace which interferes with his respiration. The same is true of shape-flow rhythms.'

There are then at least two strong lobbies for the rehabilitation (sic) of movement. Trained movement observers and analysts, particularly those adhering to some form of Effort or Effort-Shape notation, have achieved success in carefully encoding movement patterns. There is also the research base which has at the very least raised questions about social interaction. The difficulty remains, as Laban [1980, p. 17] has indicated, that: 'for a very long time man has been unable to find the connection between his movement-thinking and his word-thinking.'

Movement also has a significant role to play as an aspect of therapy. Not only can movement observation and analysis help in assessment/diagnosis, it can also be a *vehicle for treatment*. Pesso [1969, p. xii], for example, has used a system of psychomotor techniques and training which involves motor and spatial sensitization. His method 'provides a means of experiencing more of one's organic self as a living, moving organism and not only as a thinking, conceptualizing, verbalizing being'.

Pesso's system is group-based and involves three stages: sensitization to motoric impulses *(intrapsychic)*; sensitization to spatial placement *(interpersonal)*, and the handling of emotional feelings and events in 'structures' (combination of intrapsychic and interpersonal).

Reich explored the relationship between muscular tensions and emotional repression and developed a system of therapy which facilitated the release of such tension. Lowen [1971, 1976] has developed the study of bioenergetics in order 'to help a person get back together with his body'. In his exploration of 'active' therapy, Lowen [1971, p. 95] has noted: 'I wonder how much it is possible to achieve with a patient lying supine on a couch or sitting comfortably in a chair . . . the physical passivity enjoined by the prone position or the sitting position must constitute some handicap in the therapy.' In the work of Lowen and Pesso, respiration or controlled breathing plays a significant role.

Alexander brought a different approach to therapeutic practice. His systematic approach to the 'use of the self' emphasized the significance of the unity of physical and mental processes in the working of the human organism. His approach was *psychophysical* and not psychoanalytical. He was critical of some aspects of psychoanalysis as 'end-gaining' which he regarded as the: 'attempt to effect the "cure" of a specific trouble by specific means without consideration being given to the necessity of restoring a satisfactory standard of psychophysical functioning' [Barlow, 1978, p. 127ff.]. Alexander based his work on the principle that *use affects functioning* and recognized that by the time we reach adult life, if not before, most of us will have developed tension habits which are harmful. Barlow [1975, p. 18] has suggested that: 'This approach is not a fringe medicine, a neo-progressive education, a religious escape, or a quack science. It is a difficult disciplined approach to personal living which leads, through a discipline, to a personal freedom and health which is possible to some extent for most people at most ages.'

It is interesting to note that Alexander's principle is viewed by practitioners as a hypothesis and not claimed as an established, absolute truth. It offers a new way of organizing oneself.

The approaches mentioned above are examples of a range of movement. Their mode of use reflects the degree of access permitted to the therapeutic process. Many of them have arisen from a practitioner's reflection on his or her own practice. We are conscious that present-day therapy can draw upon a range of support. Our case is that where a therapist has no direct experience of movement observation, analysis and movement therapy, the inclusion of a trained movement therapist can add to the quality of therapy offered. An openness to alternatives is as we have argued fundamental to personal construct psychology and it is to this we return to conclude our discussion. Few writers in psychology have reflected on the significance of the physical modality. Salmon [1985, p. 181] has proposed an alternative reading of Kelly. She argues for a change in the metaphor of man-the-scientist: 'If we see people as embodying their experience, and as taking stances towards their lives, we can, I think, achieve a better understanding of what they do, since it is our position towards our lives which governs the kinds of engagements possible for us. Because Kelly saw inner meanings as central to human action, this redefinition of his approach may, ultimately, be truer to its essential spirit.'

The language of the body, its bearing and carriage are loaded with personal meaning. Research into the process of recognition has noted the significance of movement and underscores the importance of nonverbal socialization. As Stebbing [1984, p. 35] has suggested: 'The expression of ourselves, the experience of our world and life, are connected with physical movement, and our mental and emotional activities are bound up and inseparable from our physical freedom.'

In their conclusion to the discussion of creative arts in therapy, Feder and Feder [1981] note with some irony that the investment in dance/movement therapy brings society in a full circle. As Lowen [1971] would argue, movement therapy provides an opportunity for the person to get his/her feet 'back on the ground' literally and metaphorically.

Overprescriptive reading of Kelly, Salmon [1985] argues, has missed a fundamental aspect of personal construct theory, namely that one can know others only through knowing one's own experience. She suggests that his message is often read as: 'meaning triadic elicitation, applying elicited constructs to elements feeding the grid into a computer and inspecting the resulting statistical analyses. But, if we are really to enlarge our understanding of what is most deeply significant in our lives, perhaps we need to do something rather different from this – to pay close, careful delicate attention to our bodily selves' [p. 177].

Pope [1981] has argued that personal construct psychologists need to be more flexible in their elicitation methods and must bear the responsibility for alerting other researchers to the existence of alternative procedures. Triadic elicitation is but one approach to the elicitation of constructs. Thomas and Harri-Augstein [1985, p. 272] have pointed out, for example, that nonverbal grid games can be designed: 'to allow construers to communicate more directly without having to translate their experience into verbal irrelevancies in order to communicate. Non-verbal construing games takes one into direct contact with the texture, structure, taste, smell, form sounds and appearances of another's view of reality'.

We believe that the spirit of construct psychology invites us to explore the implications of Kelly's ideas in our own experimentation and to develop, extend and reject aspects of it. Neimeyer [1985, p. 157] has proposed that: 'If grid technique ultimately proves interesting, but too restrictive (and I believe it will), and if there are at least some seeds in Kelly's writings that deserve to be cultivated (and I think there are), then I hope that a few construct theorists will begin to explore seriously the radically different methodologies that might enable them to do so.' Neimeyer proposed several fields beyond the frontiers of psychology to which construct theorists might turn in their exploration. To his list we would add movement analysis.

In an earlier paper, Neimeyer [1981, p. 105] noted the now trivial importance of 'tacit construing' – 'all those constructs which are not verbally articulated, regardless of their point of emergence in the individuals lifespan' and pointed out that despite the fact that they 'may lack the communicability of more explicit verbal dimensions' they may, in the words of Bannister and Mair [1968, p. 29], 'occupy important and even central places in the economy of a persons orientation towards himself or the world'.

This raises an important issue. Do therapists have to facilitate verbalization of such constructs? Perhaps with sensitivity to the potential of movement, therapists can help their clients elucidate and revise such constructs in their unverbalized form through a process of creative movement.

Epting [1981, p. 193] alludes to nonverbal construing and one of the main professional tasks within therapy, i.e. the loosening and tightening of the clients construct system: 'Tightening in therapy may be illustrated by asking the client to stop and try to state exactly what was meant by a specific remark. In loosening, meaning dimensions are liberated from this kind of interlocking structure... The use of various relaxation techniques and the use of fantasy procedures would illustrate loosening in the therapeutic interview.'

Epting suggests that in loosening, preverbal constructs can become verbally labelled and then tightened in order to produce new understandings along the lines of what Kelly termed the creativity cycle. We would suggest that movement could be used *either* in a relaxation mode to loosen construing and help in articulation *or* as a means of attempting to 'state exactly' through movement. Construct psychologists and movement analysts could help clients to utilize movement as an alternative mode of communication in therapy. Arnold's [1979] book gives some pointers regarding movement vocabulary and the process of movement communication, meaning and expression.

In this chapter we have sought to explore aspects of the work of Rudolf Laban and George Kelly in a true spirit of constructive alternativism. We both have experience of dance, movement education and personal construct psychology. We have found it exciting to pursue our intuitive feelings about movement in this chapter. We recognize the paradox of writing about movement.

To our knowledge, Laban and Kelly did not meet. We hope however that by identifying aspects of their work we have indicated some epistemological similarities. We suggest that an interplay between the two offers potential for development within the context of therapy.

We end with a quote from Mordden's [1985] book, *Pooh's Workout Book*, which for us embodies constructive alternativism and the spirit with which both Kelly and Laban viewed their work:

'Why is it that you are recommending an exercise like this?' asked Piglet. 'I thought you only liked bouncy ones.'

'I guess I'm finally trying to see things your way, Piglet.'

'The best thing about it', said Pooh, 'is that instead of having to go home after the party with all the fun suddenly over, *we* get to start another party. I like that'...

References

Arnold, P.J.: Meaning in movement, sport and physical education (Heinemann, London 1979).

Bannister, D.: Issues and approaches in personal construct theory (Academic Press, London 1985).

Bannister, D.; Fransella, F.: Inquiring man; 2nd ed. (Penguin, Harmondsworth 1980).

Bannister, D.; Mair, M.: The evaluation of personal constructs (Academic Press, New York 1968).

Barfoot, J.: Gaining ground (The Women's Press, London 1980).

Barlow, W.: The Alexander principle (Arrow Books, London 1975).

Barlow, W.: More talk of Alexander (Gollancz, London 1978).

Beail, N.: Repertory grid technique and personal constructs (Croom Helm, London 1985).

Benthall, J.; Polhemus, T.: The body as a medium of expression (Allen Lane, London 1975).

Bernstein, P.L.: Theoretical approaches in dance-movement therapy, vol. 1 (Kendall/Hunt, Dubuque 1986).

Best, D.: Philosophy and human movement (Allen & Unwin, London 1978).

Birdwhistell, R.L.: Kinesics and context (Penguin, Harmondsworth, 1973).

Bodmer, S.: Memories of Laban. Laban Art Movem. Guild Mag. *63:* 7–10 (1979).

Chaiklin, S.; Schmaiss, C.: The chace approach to dance therapy; in Bernstein, Theoretical approaches to dance-movement therapy (Kendall/Hunt, Dubuque 1983).

Condon, W.S.: Linguistic-kinesic research and dance therapy. Proceedings of the Third Annual Conference of the American Dance Therapy Association (ADTA, Baltimore 1986).

Dell, C.: A primer for movement description (Dance Notation Bureau, New York 1970).

Epting, F.R.: An appraisal of personal construct psychotherapy; in Bonarius, Holland, Rosenberg, Personal construct psychology (Macmillan, London 1981).

Feder, E.; Feder, B: The expressive arts therapies (Prentice-Hall, Englewood Cliffs 1981).

Foster, R.: The analysis of movement – A current conception and the reason for it. Laban Art Movem. Guild Mag. *25:* 23–29 (1960).

Hutchinson, A.: Labanotation; 2nd ed. (Oxford University Press, London 1972).

Kelly, G.A.: The psychology of personal constructs (Norton, New York 1955).

Kelly, G.A.: Fixed role therapy: in Jurjevich, Handbook of direct and behaviour therapies (1966).

Kelly, G.A.: The strategy of psychological research; in Maher, Clinical psychology and personality: Selected papers of George Kelly (Wiley, New York 1969).

Laban, R.: Movement concerns the whole man. Laban Art Movem. Guild Mag. *21:* 9–13 (1958).

Laban, R.: A life for dance (MacDonald & Evans, London 1975).

Laban, R.: The mastery of movement; 4th ed. (MacDonald & Evans, London 1980).

Laban, R.: A vision of dynamic space (Falmer Press, London 1984).

Laban, R.; Lawrence, F.C.: Effort; 2nd ed. (MacDonald & Evans, London 1974).

Lamb, W.: Posture and gesture (Duckworth, London 1965).

Lamb, W.; Watson, E.: Body code (Routledge & Kegan Paul, London 1979).

Lowen, A.: The language of the body (Collier Books, New York 1971).

Lowen, A.: Bioenergetics (Penguin, Harmondsworth 1976).

Lyons, S.: Dance in education: A constructivist analysis; unpubl. thesis (University of Surrey 1985).

Mordden, E.: Pooh's workout book (Methuen, London 1985).

Neimeyer, R.: The structure and meaningfulness of tacit construing; in Bonarius, Holland, Rosenberg, Personal construct psychology (Macmillan, London 1981).

Neimeyer, R.: Problems and prospects in personal construct theory; in Bannister, Issues and approaches in personal construct theory (Academic Press, London 1985).

North, M.: Personality assessment through movement (MacDonald & Evans, London 1972).

Novak, J.: Constructively approaching education: toward a theory of practice. Sixth International Congress on Personal Construct Psychology. Cambridge 1985.

Patterson, C.H.: Theories of counselling and psychotherapy (Harper & Row, New York 1966).

Pesso, A.: Movement in psychotherapy (New York University Press, New York 1969).

Pope, M.: In true spirit: Constructive alternativism in educational research. Fourth International Congress on Personal Construct Psychology, Brock University, Canada 1981.

Pope, M.; Keen, T.: Personal construct psychology and education (Academic Press, London 1982).

Salmon, P.: Coming to know (Routledge & Kegan Paul, London 1980).

Salmon, P.: Relations with the physical: An alternative reading of Kelly; in Bannister, Issues and approaches in personal construct theory (Academic Press, London 1985).

Schoop, T.: Won't you join the dance? (Mayfield, Palo Alto 1974).

Skelly, M.: Developmental possibilities: A general essay. Laban Art Movem. Guild Mag. *60:* 30–40 (1978).

Stebbing, D.: The physical roots of movement: Preparing the body for action; in Warren, Using the creative arts in therapy (Croom Helm, London 1984).

Stefan, C.; Linder, H.: Suicide, an experience of chaos or fatalism: Perspectives from personal construct theory; in Bannister, Issues and approaches in personal construct theory (Academic Press, London 1985).

Thomas, L.F.; Harri-Augstein, S.: Teaching and learning as a negotiation of personal meaning; in Beail, Repertory grid technique and personal constructs (Croom Helm, London 1985).

Thornton, S.: A movement perspective of Rudolf Laban (MacDonald & Evans, London 1971).

Ullmann, L.: My apprenticeship with Laban. Laban Art Movem. Guild Mag. *63:* 21–30 (1975).

Warren, B.: Using the creative arts in therapy (Croom Helm, London 1984).

Whitehouse, M.: C.G. Jung and dance therapy: Two major principles; in Bernstein, Theoretical approaches in dance movement therapy, vol. 1 (Kendall/Hunt, Dubuque 1986).

Wigman, M.: The extraordinary thing Laban gave to the dance. Laban Art Movem. Guild Mag. *40:* 102–103 (1959).

Sue Lyons, PhD, Department of Educational Studies, University of Surrey, Guildford Surrey (UK)

Kirkcaldy B (ed): Normalities and Abnormalities in Human Movement.
Med Sport Sci. Basel, Karger, 1989, vol 29, pp 166–187

Exercise as a Therapeutic Modality

Bruce Kirkcaldy

Psychosomatic Department, University of Cologne, FRG

Introduction

Over the years, many anecdotal and observational reports have been made regarding the beneficial effects derived from participation in systematic vigorous exercise on both physical health and in the promotion of psychological well-being. Its proponents claim that exercise represents a treatment modality with unique prophylactic, rehabilitative and restorative properties.

The desirable physiological changes accompanying regular exercise appear well established, ranging from favourable *biochemical* changes (e.g. reduction in glucose and insulin levels, decrement in body fat, elevation in testosterone) through *improved physical adaptation* and *cardiovascular functioning* (e.g. larger stroke volume, lowered heart rate, reduction in blood pressure, faster physiological recovery rates, and increased aerobic capacity), to improvements in global aspects of *physical fitness* (e.g. increased strength, stamina, endurance and flexibility coupled with increased work capacity). Consequently, physically based adjunctive therapies have been commonly applied in the treatment of coronary disease, hypertension, hypokinetic diseases, metabolic disturbances, diabetes, obesity, and deficiencies of the skeletomuscular system [Beuker, 1986].

The revitalized interest in sport and exercise (body-building, 'aerobic jogging', calisthenics, and 'stretching'), propagandized by the popular media, has led to the emergence of physical exercise as an appealing and frequently prescribed variant of *psychotherapy*. Amongst the psychological benefits supposedly derived from regular, rigorous physical exercise are positive mood shifts, increased self-sufficiency, personal adjustment, enhanced body image, and improved self-concept. Moreover, physical activity appears to facilitate cognitive and perceptual processing, reduce type A (coronary-prone) behaviour, improve stress management skills and bolster perform-ance. These findings are not limited to normal populations, and exercise has been endorsed as a viable therapeutic tool in the treatment of debilitating clinical ailments, serving to alleviate *chronic depressive* disorders and ame-liorate *anxiety states*. Van Andel and Austin [1984] refer to the transposition from the central tenet of psychosomatic medicine which focuses on the impact of the mind on somatic functioning, to the somatotherapeutic pre-mise emphasizing the bodily components of the mind-body relationship in which physical activity exerts an influence on mental attitudes, inducing positive psychological states.

The empirical evidence attesting to the beneficial effects of exercise remains elusive because studies aimed at documenting the relationship be-tween physical exertion and mental health abound with methodological and statistical shortcomings, making definitive conclusions tenuous.

This article examines contemporary research in an attempt to resolve several questions. What special features characterize physical activity as a therapeutic modality? How effective does it compare to other techniques? To what extent do nonspecific factors, such as social interaction, play a role in therapeutic activity? Do individuals differ in their susceptibility to exer-cise? Who benefits least ('dropout' characteristics)? What adverse effects does rigorous physical exercise have? And, finally, what underlying mecha-nism may explain the paradoxical 'therapeutic' and 'addictive' effects of exercise?

Advantages of Therapeutic Activity

Amongst the positive features of exercise therapy are its cost-effective-ness; minimal skills or training required for its execution; in contrast to medication, it shows few undesirable side effects; client-orientedness (negligi-ble therapist intervention coupled with a high degree of activity on the part of the recipient of the treatment); prophylactic quality for reducing future mood dysfunctioning (once the therapeutic activities are known, they can be implemented at a later date without therapist support), and the dual thera-peutic character (physical and mental health benefits). Such therapies are not dependent on verbal exchange, and can thus be implemented whenever lan-guage or communicative skills are lacking or restricted, e.g. foreigners, infants, autistic children, psychotics, geriatric patients and speech-impaired. Furthermore, therapeutic gains can be monitored without professional help, e.g. the exerciser has an objective and readily amenable index of success (reduction in body weight or increase in running speed), in contrast to many therapies in which health outcome variables are vague and require professional monitoring.

Comparative Therapeutic Efficacy

Garfield [1981] provocatively suggests that '... although the different forms and types of psychotherapy emphasize their unique features and appear to vary greatly in theory, in actuality, their claims for success may be due to unemphasized factors that are common to most of them.' Generally, there are several common factors operative in most therapies. Firstly, 'hope' is available to the subject. The therapist recognizes the problems experienced, acknowledges them, expresses concern, and seeks a means of alleviating them ('offer of help'). The individual thus has an '... opportunity to ventilate feelings, to experience catharsis, and to have someone to listen to'. The client who feels motivated for a therapy program will invariably have expectations, particularly in the expertise of the therapist and the reassurance he or she offers. Finally, the therapist offers a rational explanation coupled with a novel belief system.

In order to establish whether observed psychological changes are truly attributable to exercise therapy, an adequate *control* group is required. Failure to incorporate such an *equivalent* comparison group receiving an alternative treatment schedule will, for instance, induce *positive expectations* amongst active participants, in contrast to instilling a sense of *demoralization* amongst the 'neglected' (untreated) controls.

Bahrke and Morgan [1981] attempted to evaluate the comparative efficacy of *acute* aerobic exercise and a noncultic meditative anxiolytic intervention. Seventy-five regularly exercising adult males were randomly assigned to one of three conditions; exercise, Benson's Relaxation Response (meditation), or a control group (reading a popular magazine in a sound-filtered room). The two treatment groups represent seemingly divergent procedures: physical exertion induces arousal, whereas relaxation rehearsal aims at producing quiescence. All three groups were equally effective in reducing state anxiety, and so the investigators concluded that a common element to all three conditions was the time course – the period of rest or 'time out' – which probably served to *distract* the attention of the subjects from their usual cognitive preoccupations.

A similar conclusion was reached by Greist et al. [1981] who randomly assigned patients seeking treatment for neurotic and reactive depression into one of three groups (running, time-limited psychotherapy, and time-unlimited psychotherapy) over a *10-week* period. A comparison of outcomes revealed that the somatic running treatment was equally as effective as the two traditional individual psychotherapeutic interventions in alleviating moderate depression (SCL 90) and target complaints. The running therapy appeared to make use of distractive methods, so that '... on those occasions when depressive affect and ruminations persisted during a run, the leader suggested a sequential focus on breathing, the sound and feeling of foot falls, and an awareness of the spine in an erect position.' In this manner the conversation was diverted away from the problem of depression and directed towards mechanical aspects of the running activity itself.

Lobitz et al. [1983] compared the effectiveness of physical exercise and anxiety-management training in the reduction of stress in a non-patient population. Eighteen subjects were randomly assigned to one of three groups – anxiety management, aerobic conditioning or control. The courses lasted 7 weeks. Both treatment groups yielded a significant reduction in state anxiety (STAI), and the anxiety management treatment group displayed a significant drop in trait anxiety. As expected, the aerobic exercise group revealed *unique* physiological benefits, including lowered systolic blood pressure, reduction in heart rate and increment in the high density lipoprotein, cholesterol.

Long [1984] compared the effectiveness of an aerobic 'jogging' conditioning programme with a stress inoculation training, and a waiting list control as a means of treating chronic intermittent stress. Subjects were randomly assigned to one of the three groups. Therapy sessions were of 90 min duration per week over a 10-week period, coupled with homework assignment activities. Both the stress inoculation and jogging programme participants exhibited a diminution in subjectively experienced anxiety, and improved self-efficacy, changes which persisted after cessation of the programme. Participants in the aerobic conditioning group further revealed an improvement in cardiovascular fitness.

Keller and Seraganian [1984] reported on a study to assess the effect of aerobic exercise on autonomic responsivity to psychosocial stress. Sixty subjects were randomly assigned to a group receiving 10 weeks' aerobic exercise, meditation, or music appreciation. Diverse psychosocial stressors were selected from a 6-task battery, counterbalanced across treatments and sessions. Participants in the exercise group revealed a significant improvement in physical fitness and faster electrodermal recovery rates. The authors suggested that the fast autonomic recovery which characterizes the more physically fit individual may promote *effective coping* with emotional stress.

In a study to assess the effect of aerobic conditioning and induced stress ('insoluble anagrams') on anxiety, blood pressure and muscle tension, McGlynn et al. [1983] provided a 14-week course of aerobic exercise comprising 1-hour sessions of warm-up, jogging and walking, performed twice weekly to a group of volunteers from an aerobic's class, and recruits from a health science class. After completion of the 14-week aerobic training programme, the recipients of the individualized aerobic training programme revealed a significant decrease in blood pressure, EMG activity of the biceps brachii, as well as trait and state anxiety (STAI). The control group and the conditioned group responded to the stressful situation with significantly elevated EMG activity and state anxiety, but the increase was most pronounced amongst the control group. Furthermore, the nonexercising group revealed a significant increase in blood pressure during the induced stress.

How do these effects compare with other coping techniques for managing real-life stressors? The effectiveness of exercise, social support and hardiness as resistance resources against illness amongst male business executives were compared by Kobasa et al. [1985]. Hardiness emerged as the most effective buffer providing protection against concurrent and future illness (1 year later). Exercise and social support seem to offer additional protection both concurrently and prospectively. Exercise appears *palliative* (serving a predominantly concurrent value). Its buffering effect is distinct from that attributable to the indicator, hardiness. Physical activity directly reduces the organismic strain imposed by the stressful event, without affecting the precipitating events, unlike hardiness, which represents a transformational coping strategy, decreasing the stressfulness of events.

Overall, the findings presented here are consistent with Crew and Lander's [1987] meta-analysis of 34 aerobic studies, in which 'exercise acts as a coping strategy or serves as an *inoculator* to more effectively respond to the intrusion of psychosocial stress. Exercise may provide a more efficient system for coping with psychosocial stress by reducing autonomic recovery time. As an *inoculator*, exercise training bouts may enhance the subjects' physical and psychological ability to handle stress'.

The Social Component

The majority of physical activity programmes involve a substantial *social* component. Beneficial effects assumed due to exercise may more accurately be attributable to practice of social skills, which are transferable to real-life situations. Participants in a sport recreational setting are provided with increased opportunity for group participation, social contact and acceptance within the group [Ransford, 1982].

Consider the study by Jasnoski et al. [1981]. They provided a group of females enrolled for an aerobic's course with training on a 1-hour twice-weekly basis over 10 weeks' duration. A waiting list control was available to control for potential subject selection, as well as an independent control (introductory psychology group). Individuals in the treatment condition displayed reliably greater improvements in ability and confidence in both physical and nonphysical (e.g., frustration tolerance) domains, than did controls. This indicated that perceived participation in the course had a widespread effect. Conversely, enhanced fitness levels resulting from the aerobic exercise were not related to improvement in confidence and abilities, thus indicating that not all major personal changes associated with fitness can be attributable to physical fitness changes, but seem due to other factors such as positive expectancy or participation in the group process. They suggest that 'Future research might focus on persons who are in less good physical condition for whom changes in fitness might have a greater impact, examine other psychological factors (personality traits and states), and employ more intensive training programmes. In view of the enthusiasm associated with exercise, and in view of the theoretical and practical importance of understanding the process of changing self-perception and personality, findings in this area would appear to be of wide interest and have potential for practical applications.'

In a correlational study, Schwenkmezger [1987] examined the extent that the social/situative context, rather than physical activity per se, contributes towards the attentuation of depressive symptoms. 205 subjects were required to complete a three-part inventory of attitudes towards health incorporating items related to behaviour ('I jog several times a week'), attitudes ('I think jogging is healthy'), and environment ('My friends jog regularly'). A complaints' inventory was also administered covering total complaints, psychological complaints (anxiety/phobic responses, social restraint, helplessness and depression), and physical-functional complaints (cardiorespiratory symptoms, sweating, etc.). There were low but significant correlations displayed for males between behavioural indices of physical activity and total/

physical-functional complaints, but not related to psychological symptoms. Conversely, behavioural indicators for social contact covaried more frequently and were larger with all three complaint scales, and particularly pronounced for psychological complaints. The correlations explained up to 15% of the total variance and were significant for both sexes.

Jasnoski and Holmes [1981], using the 16PF, the Self-Rating Depression Scale, and a short type A measure, have demonstrated that the initial level of aerobic fitness, aerobic training (1-hour sessions twice weekly over 15 weeks), and changes in aerobic fitness are associated with *different aspects* of psychological functioning. High initial fitness levels were related to less pretentiousness, less depression, greater self-assurance and emotional stability. Active involvement in the aerobic course was sufficient to induce positive shifts in terms of increased imagination, decreased inhibition, more self-assuredness, increased easy-goingness, and reduced coronary behaviour. An improvement in aerobic fitness was observed from pre- to posttest training. Changes in aerobic performance produced reliable personality shifts, in the direction of greater self-assuredness, less tension, and more experimenting. They concluded that physical and social factors appear to be related to different facets of personality.

An interesting social psychological explanation was proposed by Tucker [1983a] for his observation that relatively strong persons are more satisfied with their bodies and body processes, less anxious and less emotionally labile, extraverted and more confident and satisfied than less muscular persons. He comments that '... physical structure in which one resides is constantly evaluated by others as well as the self ... the strong and muscular man tends to be viewed by others as possessing more favourable skills and personality traits and tends to be perceived as more athletic and physically capable than are men with weaker constitutions' (p. 1358). The physically fit mesomorph will receive more *positive social feedback* which in turn promotes positive self-images. The author is cautious in maintaining that the correlational nature of the study does not allow causal inference; the phenomenon of selection may contribute to the personality-strength relationship, so that males with healthy personalities may train more physically.

The Dropout

Even in instances where exercise has been demonstrated as an effective treatment modality, participants do not necessarily adhere to the programme. The loss of subjects ('attrition') is a major threat to the internal validity of studies which implement therapeutic intervention. Studies in which the dropout rate is high reduces the clinical trial to a prospective study, making generalizability from compliers to noncompleters impossible.

In a recent study, Shephard et al. [1986] claim that 'even with the convenience of well-designed and heavily funded experimental classes in the work place, the initial participation rate is typically no more than 20% of eligible individuals'.

A review of the literature indicated that *about 35%* of the subjects in *cardiac rehabilitation* programmes will drop out within 6 months of entry. The potential noncomplier was identified as likely to be *inactive* in his leisure time, type A in behaviour, a *smoker*, a *blue-collar* worker, and have had *more than one infarction* [Oldbridge, 1981] – features which suggest they are less 'health conscious'. In a study by Gale et al. [1984], involving a 6-month exercise schedule, early dropouts (< 10% of programme attendance) were inclined to display low self-motivation (males only), *less stability* in the community (short residence, frequent change of address, or short job tenure), be *single* rather than married, have *no children*, and be *more* physically fit (insufficient challenge?).

Blumenthal et al. [1982] documented the rates of noncompliance on a 1-year cardiac rehabilitation aerobic exercise scheme amongst patients recovering from myocardial infarction compared to prospectively determined baseline scores. Compliers were defined as those who attended at least 75% of the scheduled sessions. Forty percent of the subjects 'dropped out' and these were characterized by MMPI psychological profiles as *more depressed, hypochondriacal, socially introverted, anxious* and *lower in ego strength* compared to the completers. The compliers were, additionally, *more defensive* (L and K scores were significantly higher). These psychological variables were associated with noncompliance *independently* of physical status (extent of myocardial damage prior to infarction).

Dishman [1981] reports on a prospective study examining psychosocial factors implicated in adherence. Sixty-six adult males participated 3 days per week over a period of 20 weeks in organized exercise involving muscular or cardiovascular endurance training. Dropouts and compliers were effectively discriminated on the basis of their *body weight, self-motivation* and *percent body fat*. By identifying such drop-out susceptible individuals, it may be possible to promote health education strategies designed to facilitate adherence and Dishman conjectures that '... since self-motivation assessment is based upon self-perceptions of perseverant behaviour, it is theoretically possible that this construct might be altered as a function of an exercise experience. In this regard, an individual who initially possesses low self-motivation but who is somehow able to maintain involvement beyond what appears to be the critical 3–5 month period may subsequently make a self-attribution of increased self-motivation, which might then perpetuate adherence independent of further administrative intervention'.

The identification of dropout characteristics clearly does not offer an *explanatory* account of attrition. An attempt to introduce a theoretical construct relevant to the problem was provided by McCready and Long [1985]. They examined the relationship between the combined effects of locus of control and attitudes towards physical activity and exercise adherence. Sixty-one female volunteer recruits participated in an 8-to-12-week aerobic exercise programme designed to increase cardiovascular endurance, flexibility, strength, movement control and body awareness. A weak relationship existed between adherence and the locus and attitude scales. A stepwise regression revealed that those persons who at the beginning of the programme displayed a more *positive attitude toward involvement as a means of reducing stress and tension*, and a less positive attitude toward exercise participation for continuing social relations, were likely to demonstrate higher attendance rates. Shephard et al. [1986] also propose that '... there may indeed be value in attempting to shape attitudes and beliefs before inviting the uncommitted to engage in significant exercise behaviour'.

Andrew et al. [1981] focused on social determinants of dropout behaviour from a large-scale 7-year exercise regimens programme with postcoronary patients. These long-term programmes assigned subjects randomly to a low intensity or high intensity (designed to maximize a training response) group. The responses to a psychosocial questionnaire were compared using χ^2 analysis to determine significant classes of questions and subsequently, a logistic transform model was used to isolate those specific items which were associated with rate of noncompliance. The three main categories which affected dropout rate were: *perception of the programme, family and life-style*, and *convenience factors* of the exercise centre. The authors suggest that long-term rehabilitation trials ought to consider such social constraints in order to optimize compliance.

Diverse intervention techniques have been applied, e.g. positive reinforcement and self-control, as a means of ensuring maintenance of exercise. An attempt was made by Atkins et al. [1984] to evaluate behavioural and cognitive-behavioural programmes for increasing compliance rates in the management of chronic obstructive pulmonary disease (COPD) using a walking exercise prescription. The COPD patients were randomly assigned to one of five experimental treatments (cognitive modification, behavioural modification, cognitive-behavioural modification, attention control and a no-treatment control – the latter group was provided with an exercise prescription, but received no training on implementation). The three treated groups displayed increases in exercise over the initial 3 months compared to the no-treatment group. *'Cognitive-behaviour' strategies* demonstrated the highest compliance rates of all groups. All three treatment groups revealed a substantial improvement in their exercise tolerance, General Health Status Index ('quality of well-being') and self-efficacy in comparison to the non-treatment groups.

There are obvious limitations to such studies involving predominantly cardiovascular patients: More studies are required assessing 'early dropout' and 'long-term maintenance of training' in other clinical populations, e.g. depressives and neurotics. Nevertheless, several recommendations were outlined by Martin and Dubbert [1982] for promoting maintenance of exercise in a comprehensive evaluation of the literature (in which subject, social-environmental, and exercise programme factors were examined for diverse medical ailments, e.g. cardiovascular risk, obesity, and diabetes) in which '... the optimal treatment package should probably include a very convenient location (e.g. neighbourhood-based programs), group-based, lower intensity exercise with enthusiastic participant therapists, ample modeling, feedback and social reinforcement, flexible, participant-influenced exercise goal-setting, and extensive family/social involvement'.

Differential Therapeutic Outcomes

Clinical studies evaluating therapeutic effectiveness frequently assume that patient samples represent homogeneous collectives. Such suppositions are invalid. Subjects do in fact display considerable variation in their responsivity to therapies; further, therapeutic gains can be optimized if treatment modalities are selected compatible with an individual's requirements.

This is well illustrated in such mental health parameters as anxiety, which is a multicomponential rather than a global, unidimensional construct. The differential outcome of exercise was witnessed in a study by Schwartz et al. [1978], in which physical activity was an effective therapeutic tool in the relief of *somatic* ('emotionality') rather than cognitive ('worry' or task-irrelevant cognitions) anxiety. Similar results were obtained in

Long's [1985] 15-month follow-up study comparing the effectiveness of aerobic conditioning with stress inoculation training in the alleviation of anxiety in chronically stressed subjects. Reports of reduced anxiety and greater efficacy were maintained at the follow-up phase. Individuals displaying prevalently cognitive anxiety were inclined to show no change or an increase in anxiety from the post-to follow-up session, whereas those experiencing stress as essentially *somatic* anxiety continued to display a reduction in anxiety level.

In monitoring cardiovascular patterns corresponding to different emotional states following imagery and exercise, Schwartz et al. [1981] had found that exercise in an angry mental state evinced distinctly different cardiovascular demands than when exercising in a normal or relaxed state. Such findings may explain the beneficial recuperative effects that aerobic jogging has for some sufferers of cardiovascular disease, whilst functioning adversely for others. Type A and B running may be quite different. Emotional states were shown to influence more than movement rate. Anger yielded a different cardiovascular response pattern from fear and happiness, whereas sadness (systolic pressure and heart rate were almost as high as when exercising) differed from relaxation, despite comparable movement rates.

Congruent with these findings, Blumenthal et al. [1980] found that in a sample of middle-aged adults free from cardiovascular disease, both type A and B subjects displayed a reduction in coronary risk factors after 10 weeks' supervised exercise, but only type A individuals demonstrated lowered Jenkin Activity Survey Scores.

The relationship between regular aerobic exercise and stress tolerance was examined, in a realistic racing context, by Dienstbier et al. [1981]. Of particular interest were the individual differences which emerged along the variable, level of *commitment to running*. Persons who were highly committed, displayed substantial reductions in fear and anxiety on transition from the nonrun to short-run condition, with no change being observed from the short-run to marathon. Similarly, a dramatic decrease in capillary constriction and galvanic skin response was observed amongst the highly committed runners. In spite of the reductions found in both groups for the psychological and physiological stress indicators from the no-run to short-run phase, larger and more consistent improvements were obtained for those persons who felt highly committed to running.

Tucker [1983b] evaluated the effects of a twice-weekly training with weights over a 16-week term, on self-concept of college males. The treatment group was compared to a control receiving educational training on personal health topics. Significant posttest differences emerged in global, internal, and external self-concept between groups, substantiating the proposition that regular training is positively related to an improvement of self-concept. *Pretest trait neuroticism, self-concept*, and *body cathexis* were potent predictors of global self-concept change from initial to posttest. The author concludes that '... males who display relatively low body cathexis or self-concept scores or relatively high neuroticism characteristics at the outset of training tend to experience significantly more improvement in global self-concept than do lifters who deviate from such a psychological profile'. It is suggested that '... future investigations must seek not only to determine *if* exercise enhances psychological well-being, but research must be designed to confront the important issues of *who* tends to benefit most from *what* types of activity and *why*' (p. 396).

Similarly, Eickhoff et al. [1983] observed that chronic participation in aerobic exercise coincided with a reduction in resting heart rate and SSF (sum of skinfolds taken over several different locations, e.g. triceps, midaxillar, and abdominal), as well as an improvement along psychological variables, level of self-esteem, and self-perception of body and state of health. The benefits appeared limited, however, to those women who exhibited inferior fitness levels *prior to* commencement of the moderate intensity conditioning programme.

To summarize, the benefits of exercise are most apparent for those persons with low initial fitness, low body concept and cathexis, high neuroticism, and body-focussed anxiety. The improvement in mental health is partly attributable to a regression effect. In addition, however, there is evidence that the impact of exercise is *nonlinearly* related to psychological well-being. Physical activity serves a therapeutic function when psychological tension is coupled with low activity/sedentary life-styles. Conversely, excessive physical exertion may bring about a deterioration in psychological and physical health. The next section examines this premise.

Adverse Effects of Exercise

There are indications that exercise is not necessarily health-promoting, and indeed may be contraindicated. The proponents of regular exercise have referred to the positive addictive features of compulsive exercise, characterized by a loss of sense of self, euphoria, and total integration. In contrast, 'exercise-dependent' individuals may show characteristics of *negative addic-*

tion when prevented from exercising. Some of the most frequently observed symptoms of negative addiction include lapses in attention, an inability to concentrate, distorted self-image, restlessness, feelings of guilt, tension and anxiety, fatigue and rigidity of dietary habits. Other adverse effects of excessive exercise such as 'jogger's nipples, runner's trots, jogger's hematuria, stress fractures and anecdotal deleterious effects on family and friends cannot be ignored' [Appenzeller, 1981].

The phenomenon of exercise *addiction* amongst runners has been the focus of several studies. Glasser [1976] found that a short interruption in running induced symptoms akin to *drug withdrawal*, such as hostility, headache, frustration, and tension. Similarly, Robbins and Joseph [1985] examined the type and frequency of sensations which are experienced by runners of varied mileage, after exercise withdrawal. The predominant experiences were associated with adverse *emotional-psychological* feeling states (restlessness, frustration, irritability, and guilt) as opposed to psycho-physiological complaints (insomnia, digestive difficulties and muscle tension) – not fully consistent with the findings of Schwartz et al. [1978] in which exercise alleviated body-localized anxiety. Runners were inclined to run for longer periods as a means of avoiding the adverse sensations resulting from abstinence of physical activity: an increase in mileage, however, did not always produce more frequent stressful experiences when running had been withheld. The authors are critical themselves of their measures of deprivation, the latter based on *retrospective* self-reports (contaminated by incorrect recall) of frequency, rather than intensity of sensations.

Crossman et al. [1987] found no evidence of unpleasant effects of short-term abstinence from physical training amongst a group of swimmers and runners. In fact, despite frequent reports of addiction by athletes, they generally exhibited positive mood shifts during the day-off, suggesting a release from tension associated with training. In both sports, males and top-class athletes displayed more negative moods ('addiction pattern') during lay-off, compared to females and participants at lower classes of competitive involvement ('relief pattern'). The authors suggest that the manner in which athletes react to *short-term lay-off* may be influenced by two opposing mechanisms – negative effects as a consequence of exercise withdrawal, and positive mood changes resulting from dissipation of the fatigue which accumulates through overtraining. The authors correctly warn about the difficulties generalizing these results: the investigation constitutes a quasi-experimental design in which lay-off may have been implemented for reasons other than the investigation.

What evidence is there for psychopathological attributes amongst persistent runners? It has been suggested that habitual exercise enthusiasts exhibit behaviour similar to sufferers of anorexia nervosa (hyperactivity, heightened anxiety associated with distorted constructs of body image, and excessively rigid dietary repertoires). Wheeler et al. [1986] conducted a cross-sectional study involving 31 high- and 18 low-mileage, and 18 sedentary males. The high-mileage group (> 40 miles/week) scored significantly higher on both energy level and infrequency scores of the Jackson Personality Inventory, but showed no evidence of psychopathology. Runners showed no signs of anoxeria nervosa as indexed by the Eating Attitudes Test, but high-mileage runners did reveal a *slight* distortion of body image shown in the tendency to overestimate waist size, probably reflecting an undue concern about their figure. These findings are consistent with a recent investigation by Weight and Noakes [1987] who observed that abnormal eating attitudes and frequency of anorexia nervosa were not common amongst female athletes. Amongst the more *competitive* and *successful* athletes, however, there was an increased likelihood of psychological and physical features of anorexia nervosa.

In addition to the above-mentioned psychological problems associated with withdrawal, excessive indulgence in sport has been shown to lead to a disturbingly high rate of *muscular injuries* as observed by Kavanagh and Shephard [1977] in a group of averagely endowed middle-aged and elderly track competitors who had faithfully adhered to an arduous endurance training regimen of up to 40 miles/week into advancing age.

Is injury related to personality? Physical injuries amongst compulsive runners, who had been running for an average of 5 years, was addressed in an investigation by Diekhoff [1984]. Subjects were assessed on personal compulsivity, running-produced injuries, and training style. Each of the compulsivity measures correlated with different injury measures; 'type A–B' with 'reported injuries', 'commitment to running' with 'use of physical therapy or drugs', and 'addiction to running' with 'visits to the doctor'. Of the training variables, 'weekly mileage', 'average running length', and 'participation in fun runs and races' were related to injury variables as well; partialling out differences in training style did not appreciably affect the compulsivity-injury relationship. Those athletes categorized as injured runners were inclined to be addicted to running, type A, participants over longer distances, more committed to running, and involved in more races than noninjured runners. Diekhoff cautions about inferences drawn in the study, since the personality-injury relationship was explored *after* the injury had occurred.

Zuckerman [1983] also demonstrated that psychological variables may be important in predicting athletic injury. Sensation-seeking, a personality trait with descriptive features similar to type A behaviour, was related to those sporting pursuits involving novel sensations and risk-taking, a relationship which was particularly strong for experienced athletes. High sensation-seekers tend to be reckless, underestimating the risk associated with certain sports. Consequently, they exhibit higher injury rates, in contrast to low sensation-seekers who avoid high risk activities such as hang-gliding, mountaineering, parachuting or scuba-diving. Fear of injury was reported to be negatively correlated with sensation-seeking.

Problems in generalizability are likely in studies relying on such selective samples, e.g. athletes represent a special population, high on need for achievement, competitive drive and values attached to physical activity. In a study by Little [1981], neurotics were dichotomized along the extremes of a dimension of personal valued athleticism/physical prowess. For non-athletic (male) neurotics it is rare that physical threat induces neurotic symptomatology since physical ability is not particularly highly rated, in contrast to neurotics displaying athletic personalities for whom direct threat to one's physical well-being ('physical assault') precipitates neurotic (deprivation) breakdown when compared to nonathletic male neurotics. The neurotic athletic types were characterized by a relative absence of neurotic incidents in their early life history, minimal psychiatric and physical morbidity within family history, and satisfactory personal relationships. 'Psychometrically' they were significantly more *extraverted* and more *emotionally stable*, differences which could not be attributed to age differences. Little [1981] comments that '... even excessive athleticism is not in itself neurotic ... like exclusive and excessive emotional dependence on work, on family relationship bonds, intellectual pursuits, physical beauty, sexual prowess or any other overvalued attribute or activity, athleticism can place the subject in a vulnerable preneurotic state leading to manifest neurotic illness in the event of an *appropriate* threat, or actual enforced deprivation especially if abrupt or unexpected'.

The Endorphin Connection

What physiological mechanism underlies the favourable mood shifts, pain-reducing effects, as well as the adverse changes, e.g. 'addiction', associated with rigorous physical activity?

The endogenous opiates may constitute the biochemical basis for negative addiction. These endogenous neurotransmitters, enkephalin and the associated endorphins, are morphine-like peptides. They appear to modulate mood states, induce euphoria, and possess analgesic properties. It has been shown that negative affective states result from a deficiency of these opiate-like substances within the central nervous system, particularly the hypophysis. Since vigorous physical activity appears to elevate the level of opioid beta-endorphin concentrations, implementation of somatomotor exercise therapy may reduce anxiety and enhance mood states.

A couple of studies run counter to the 'endorphin-mediated mood hypothesis'. Markoff et al. [1982] observed a reduction in anger-hostility and tension-anxiety amongst marathoners after running for an hour at a customary training pace. Naloxone, a narcotic antagonist, failed to reverse the mood shift when given subcutaneously (in a double-blind and counterbalanced study), suggesting that endorphins did not mediate mood changes. Similarly, William and Getty [1986] found that subjects in an aerobic exercise class produced a substantial improvement in cardiovascular functioning, without altering psychological mood state (compared to a placebo control and group of nonexercisers). The basal plasma levels of beta-endorphins amongst the depressed subjects did not appear related to physical activity. These results are consistent with those obtained by Goldfarb et al. [1987] who analysed the effects of graded exercise testing to exhaustion, on serum beta-endorphin levels. Untrained males were required to exercise up to maximum capacity on an ergometer. Exercise did produce a significant increase in beta-endorphin levels but the correlation observed between exercise *intensity* and the level of serum beta-endorphin was not significant (0.30).

Diverse studies have indicated that the relationship between endorphins and physical activity is moderated by the intensity of the exercise. For instance, Hollmann et al. [1986] reported that the concentrations of adrenocorticotropin (ACTH) and beta-endorphins in peripheral blood remained unchanged during a 1-hour bout of submaximal exercise on a bicycle ergometer at below the anaerobic threshold, whereas lactic acid concentrations increased moderately and levelled off. At *maximal work rate* both ACTH and beta-endorphin levels revealed a significant increase as was the case for lactic acid. The levels of these hormones and lactic acid continued to rise 5 min after cessation of exercise. Although a decrement was observed 20 min after exercise, the values were in excess of the pre-exercise levels.

Consistent with the previous study, Rahkila et al. [1987] reported that experienced endurance athletes yielded increases in the plasma concentrations of endorphins and 'ACTH' in response to strenuous (treadmill) exercise, whereas submaximal exercise (outdoor running) did not elicit a significant metabolic response. Grossman and Sutton [1985] claim that endorphins appear to exert a negligible effect on the cardiovascular response to exercise, except during *intense* exercise, when they serve to partly inhibit ventilatory responses to physical exertion; the increased opiate activity in trained athletes resulting in lower ventilation rates is likely to be accompanied by reduced respiratory muscle fatigue at high work rate.

The importance of controlling for (naloxone) dosage is underlined in a study by Haier et al. [1981] who investigated subjectively reported pain threshold amongst a group of 15 volunteers, habitual runners, accustomed to training over an average of 21 miles/week. After assessing baseline perceived pain ratings – using standard weights applied to the finger – participants were injected either with a placebo or a 2-mg dosage of naloxone. Pain receptivity was recorded after a 1-mile run. The naloxone trial which was intended to partially block or inhibit the endorphin response 'paradoxically' produced a significant increment in the ability to withstand pain (gain in threshold time), in contrast to the placebo which produced a nonsignificant increase. An attempt to replicate these results with a larger dosage (10 mg) reversed these findings; naxolone inhibited the analgesic effect, and a gain in pain threshold was displayed by the placebo.

What further evidence is there that the *physiological dependency* on endorphins may underlay the negative symptoms of withdrawal, and adverse effects of intensive physical activity? In an earlier investigation, Farrell et al. [1982] concluded that: 'The increased levels of Bh-Ep/Bh-LPH (beta-endorphin and lipoprotein) found in this study immediately after exercise suggest that a runner who trains on a regular basis may produce endogenous opiates, which could lead to a desire for more running. The pattern of running habits commonly seen by the investigators is that runners tend to run faster and more frequently as they become experienced. These observations are not dissimilar to the development of tolerance to addictive drugs... (as) exercisers may become psychologically dependent or *addicted* to exercise.' Furthermore, it may be that the reduction in pain sensitivity during vigorous bodily exertion underlies the high injury rate observed amongst 'addicted' athletes.

Conclusions and Implications

Regular physical exertion emerges as a comparatively effective means of coping with stress. The psychological benefits are statistically and clinically significant, and are found across diverse laboratory psychosocial stressors, real-life stressors, and instances of clinical anxiety/depression. Multiple indicators reveal that the positive shifts are witnessed at a variety of levels (convergent validity) such as subjective reports, knowledgeable informant ratings, and at a physiological level. Since physical activities differ in terms of physiological, social and psychological components, various nonspecific programme factors, such as opportunity for social interaction, distraction from cognitive stressors, and increased bodily awareness, may contribute to the positive psychological shifts observed.

Individuals differ in their 'susceptibility' to different types of treatment. Van Andel and Austin [1984] emphasize the need to individualize exercise regimens to fulfil the specific requirements of subjects. Personality, self-perception, physical condition, and values held towards physical attitudes influence the therapeutic efficacy (as do differences in therapists' communication skills and experience [Greist et al., 1981]). For instance, anxious individuals displaying disorders of a somatic character profit most from therapeutic activity (in contrast to relaxation, meditation and self-awareness programmes, which are more tailored for cognitive anxiety states), as do persons displaying a low body concept and inferior physical condition. On the basis of the findings of Blumenthal et al. [1982], social extraverts are inclined to gravitate more towards *group recreational* activities, reaping more benefits from social interaction, in contrast to introverts who feel threatened from such 'gatherings'. For this reason, solitary exercise may be more suited for socially inhibited individuals.

Programme characteristics, such as convenience and family support, are important determinants of *beginning* a physical activity regimens, and the '... health and physical educator would be wise to emphasize factors which relate to perceived barriers. After such perceived barriers as lack of time, family or job responsibilities and so forth are identified, the health professional can proceed to suggest ways to overcome them. Examples of such strategies might include advice on how to elicit family or employer support for time spent jogging or exercising, or a discussion of time-management techniques which will allow individuals to fit exercise into their lives' [Slenker et al., 1984].

Failure to *comply* with a long-term, rigorously structured exercise programme destroys equivalence of groups established through randomization. At a practical level, dropout presents a costly health problem, and implies that recalcitrant patients are often left untreated. By identifying the potential dropout early in the training programme, it may be possible to implement techniques promptly for increasing adherence. In addition to personality and attitudinal factors, motivation appears to play a major role in the maintenance of exercise, so that, for '... long-term trials where the treatment outcome may be slow to develop, it is essential that the participant's motivation to maintain the health behaviour change be kept as high as possible' [Andrew et al., 1981]. This can be achieved by using cognitive and behavioural methods of reinforcement. Other methods of increasing compliance would be by altering the structure and form of the programme to take account of personal needs.

Positive affect and physical activity appear to be curvilinearly related. It is evident that whereas moderate increases in exercise improve physical health and psychological well-being, too much exercise ('neurotic athlete') may have deleterious effects. Excessive, 'compulsive' exercise appears to share features akin to negative addiction, as well as increasing risk of physical injury. Traits such as sensation-seeking, type A, and risk-taking appear implicated in the rate of physical injury.

Finally, there is a need for elucidation of the underlying mechanism which explains apparently paradoxical phenomena such as positive mood changes, negative addiction and increased injury rate. The endogenous opioids are good 'candidates'; both serum beta-endorphin and beta-lipotrophin levels increase substantially with exercise and these morphine-like substances appear to modulate mood states and pain receptivity, and have been shown to correlate significantly with trait and state anxiety. The findings are provocative, however, and despite refinements in the techniques available for locating these natural opioids, Ransford [1982] has warned that searches for single transmitter substances are likely to be 'premature and oversimplified'.

References

Andrew, G.M.; Oldbridge, N.B.; Parker, J.O.; Cunningham, D.A.; Rechnitzer, P.A.; Jones, N.L.; Buck, C.; Kavanagh, T.; Shephard, R.J.; Sutton, J.R.; McDonald, W.: Reasons for dropout from exercise programs in post-coronary patients. Med. Sci. Sports Exerc. *13:* 164–168 (1981).

Appenzeller, O.: What makes us run? New Eng. J. Med. *305:* 578–579 (1981).

Atkins, C.J.; Kaplan, R.M.; Timms, R.M.; Reinsch, S.; Lofback, K.: Behavioural exercise programs in the management of chronic obstructive pulmonary disease. J. consult. clin. Psychol. *52:* 591–603 (1984).

Bahrke, M.S.; Morgan, W.P.: Anxiety reduction following exercise and meditation; in Sacks, Sachs, Psychology of running (Kinetics Publishers, Champaign 1981).

Beuker, F.: Wer Sport treibt, lebt gesünder. Erkenntnisse präventiver Sportmedizin; in Franke, Sport und Gesundheit (Sport and health) (Rowohlt, Reinbeck bei Hamburg 1986).

Blumenthal, J.A.; Williams, R.S.; Wallace, A.G.; Williams, R.B.; Needles, T.L.: Physiological and psychological variables predict compliance to prescribed exercise therapy in patients recovering from myocardial infarction. Psychosom. Med. *44:* 519–527 (1982).

Blumenthal, J.A.; Williams, R.S.; Williams, R.B.; Wallace, A.G.: Effects of exercise on the type A (coronary-prone) behaviour pattern. Psychosom. Med. *42:* 289–296 (1980).

Crews, D.J.; Landers, D.M.: A metaanalysis review of aerobic fitness and reactivity to psychosocial stressors. Med. Sci. Sports Exerc. *19:* 114–120 (1987).

Crossman, J.; Jamieson, J.; Henderson, L.: Responses of competitive athletes to lay-offs in training: Exercise addiction or psychological relief? J. Sport Behav. *10:* 28–38 (1987).

Diekhoff, G.M.: Running amok: Injuries in compulsive runners. J. Sport Behav. *7:* 120–129 (1984).

Dienstbier, R.A.; Crabbe, J.; Johnson, G.O.; Thorland, W.; Jorgensen, J.A.; Sadar, M.M.; LaVelle, D.C.: Exercise and stress tolerance; in Sacks, Sachs, Psychology of running (Kinetics Publishers, Champaign 1981).

Dishman, R.K.: Prediction of adherence to habitual physical activity; in Nagle, Montoye, Exercise in health and disease (Thomas, Springfield 1981).

Eickhoff, J.; Thorland, W.; Ansorge, C.: Selected phsyiological and psychological effects of aerobic dancing among young adult women. J. Sports Med. *23:* 273–280 (1983).

Farrell, P.A.; Gates, W.K.; Maksud, M.G.; Morgan, W.P.: Increases in plasma beta-endorphin/ beta-lipotropin immunoreactivity after treadmill running in humans. J. appl. Physiol. *52:* 1245–1249 (1982).

Gale, J.B.; Eckhoff, W.T.; Mogel, S.F.; Rodnick, J.E.: Factors related to adherence to an exercise program for healthy adults. Med. Sci. Sports Exerc. *16:* 544–549 (1984).

Garfield, S.L.: Critical issues in the effectiveness of psychotherapy; in Walker, Clinical practice of psychology (Pergamon Press, Oxford 1981).

Glasser, W.: Positive addiction (Harper & Row, New York 1976).

Goldfarb, A.H.; Hatfield, B.D.; Sforzo, G.A.; Flynn, M.G.: Serum beta-endorphin levels during a graded exercise test to exhaustion. Med. Sci. Sport Med. *91:* 78–82 (1987).

Greist, J.H.; Klein, M.H.; Eischens, R.R.; Faris, J.; Gurman, A.S.; Morgan, W.P.: Running through your mind; in Sacks, Sachs, Psychology of running (Kinetics Publishers, Champaign 1981).

Grossman, A.; Sutton, J.R.: Endorphins; What are they? How are they measured? What is their role in exercise? Med. Sci. Sports Med. *171:* 74–81 (1985).

Haier, R.K.; Quaid, K.; Mills, J.S.C.: Naloxone alters pain perception after jogging. Psychiat. Res. *5:* 231–232 (1981).

Hayden, R.M.; Allen, G.J.: Relationship between aerobic exercise, anxiety, and depression: Convergent validation by knowledgeable informants. J. Sports Med. *24:* 69–74 (1984).

Hollmann, W.; Rost, R.; De Meirleir, K.; Liesen, H.; Heck, H.; Mader, A.: Cardiovascular effects of extreme physical training. Acta med. scand., suppl. 711, pp. 193–203 (1986).

Jasnoski, M.L.; Holmes, M.L.: Influence of initial aerobic fitness, aerobic training and changes in aerobic fitness on personality functioning. J. psychosom. Res. *25:* 553–556 (1981).

Jasnoski, M.L.; Holmes, D.S.; Solomon, S.; Aguiar, C.: Exercise, changes in aerobic capacity, and changes in self-perceptions: An experimental investigation. J. Res. Personal *15:* 460–466 (1981).

Kavanagh, T.; Shephard, R.J.: The effects of continued training on the aging process. Ann. N.Y. Acad. *301:* 656–670 (1977).

Keller, S.; Seraganian, P.: Physical fitness level and autonomic reactivity to psychosocial stress. J. psychosom. Res. *28:* 279–287 (1984).

Kobasa, S.C.O.; Maddi, S.R.; Puccetti, M.C.; Zola, M.A.: Effectiveness of hardiness, exercise and social support as resources against illness. J. psychosom. Res. *29:* 525–533 (1985).

Little, J.C.: The athlete's neurosis – a deprivation crisis; in Sacks, Sachs, Psychology of running (Kinetics Publishers, Champaign 1981).

Lobitz, W.C.; Brammell, H.L.; Stoll, S.; Niccoli, A.: Physical exercise and anxiety management training for cardiac stress management in a nonpatient population. J. card. Rehabil. *3:* 683–688 (1983).

Long, B.C.: Aerobic conditioning and stress inoculation: A comparison of stress-management interventions. Cogn. Ther. Res. *8:* 517–542 (1984).

Long, B.C.: Stress-management interventions: A 15-month follow-up of aerobic conditioning and stress inoculation training. Cogn. Ther. Res. *9:* 471–478 (1985).

Markoff, R.A.; Ryan, P.; Young, T.: Endorphins and mood changes in long-distance running. Med. Sci. Sports Exerc. *14:* 11–15 (1982).

Martin, J.E.; Dubbert, P.M.: Exercise applications and promotion in behavioural medicine: Current status and future directions. J. consult. clin. Psychol. *50:* 1004–1017 (1982).

McCready, M.L.; Long, B.C.: Locus of control, attitudes towards physical activity, and exercise adherence. J. Sport Psychol. *7:* 346–359 (1985).

McGlynn, G.H.; Franklin, B.; Lauro, G.; McGlynn, I.K.: The effect of aerobic conditioning and induced stress on state-trait anxiety, blood pressure, and muscle tension. J. Sports Med. *23:* 341–351 (1983).

Oldbridge, N.B.: Dropout and potential compliance – improving strategies in exercise rehabilitation; in Nagle, Montoye, Exercise in health and disease (Thomas, Springfield 1981).

Rahkila, P.; Hakala, E.; Salminen, K.; Laatkainen, T.: Response of plasma endorphins to running exercises in male and female endurance athletes. Med. Sci. Sport Exerc. *19:* 451–455 (1987).

Ransford, C.P.: A role of amines in the antidepressant effect of exercise: A review. Med. Sci. Sports Med. *14:* 1–10 (1982).

Robbins, J.M.; Joseph, P.: Experiencing exercise withdrawal: Possible consequences of therapeutic and mastery running. Sport Psychol. *7:* 23–39 (1985).

Schwartz, G.E.; Davidson, R.J.; Goleman, D.J.: Patterning of cognitive and somatic processes in the self-regulation of anxiety: Effects of meditation vs. exercise. Psychosom. Med. *40:* 321–328 (1978).

Schwartz, G.E.; Weinberger, D.A.; Singer, J.A.: Cardiovascular differentiation of happiness, sadness, anger, and fear following imagery and exercise. Psychosom. Med. *43:* 343–364 (1981).

Schwenkmezger, P.: Sport and therapy (unpubl. manuscript, 1987).

Shephard, R.J., Montelpare, W.; Berridge, M.; Flowers, J.: Influence of exercise and of lifestyle education upon attitudes to exercise of older people. J. Sports Med. *26:* 175–179 (1986).

Slenker, S.E.; Price, J.H.; Roberts, S.M.; Jurs, S.G.: Joggers vs. non-joggers: An analysis of knowledge, attitudes and beliefs about jogging. Res. Q. Exercise Sport *55:* 371–370 (1984).

Tucker, L.A.: Muscular strength and mental health. J. personal. soc. Psychol. *45:* 1355–1360 (1983a).

Tucker, L.A.: Effect of weight training on self-concept: A profile of those influenced most. Res. Q. Exercise Sport *4:* 389–397 (1983b).

Van Andel, G.E.; Austin, D.R.: Physical fitness and mental health: A review of the literature. Adapted Physical Activity Q. *1:* 201–220 (1984).

Weight, L.M.; Noakes, T.D.: Is running an analog of anorexia? A survey of the incidence of eating disorders in female distance runners. Med. Sci. Sport Exerc. *19:* 213–217 (1987).

Wheeler, G.D.; Wall, S.R.; Belcastro, A.N.; Conger, P.; Cumming, D.C.: Are anorexic tendencies prevalent in the habitual runner? Br. J. Sports Med. *20:* 77–81 (1986).

William, J.E.; Getty, D.: Effect of levels of exercise on psychological mood states, physical fitness, and plasma beta-endorphin. Percept. Mot. Skills *63:* 1099–1105 (1986).

Zuckerman, M.: Sensation-seeking and sports. Personal. Individ. Diff. *4:* 285–293 (1983).

Bruce Kirkcaldy, Dr. phil., Psychosomatische Abteilung, Universitätskliniken Köln, Joseph-Stelzmann-Strasse 9, D–5000 Köln (FRG)

Kirkcaldy B (ed): Normalities and Abnormalities in Human Movement.
Med Sport Sci. Basel, Karger, 1989, vol 29, pp 188–208

Movement Skills and Social Skills Training

Adrian Furnham

Department of Psychology, University College, London, UK

Introduction

One of the most popular forms of 'psychological' therapy practised in a wide range of settings and with a wide variety of patients is social skills training (SST). SST has been performed in schools, prisons, mental hospitals, outpatient clinics with patients or clients including schizophrenics [Wallace et al., 1980], neurotics [Argyle et al., 1974], criminals and delinquents [Spence and Marzillier, 1981], alcoholics and drug addicts [Oei and Jackson, 1980], as well as children and adolescents [Furnham, 1986], professional groups [Pendleton and Furnham, 1980] and handicapped individuals [Gresham, 1981].

In order to understand how movement skills are an integral part of SST, it is first necessary to deal, albeit in brief, with the history of SST and thence the theory behind the therapy. As will be shown, both have interesting problems which means that there is considerable diversity in the definition and practice of SST. Furthermore, recent developments in the area have moved far away from the original conception so that for some practitioners very little emphasis is placed on movement skills and most on cognitive strategies.

A Brief History

Furnham [1985] has pointed out some of the major differences between the history of SST in America and Europe. However, what links the original two approaches is their behaviouristic base in the sense that both were originally interested almost exclusively in social behaviour and to a far lesser degree in social cognition.

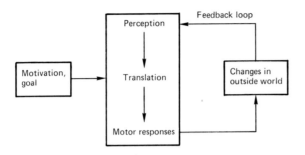

Fig. 1. Motor skill model.

In Great Britain, SST emerged out of applied occupational psychology [Welford, 1981]. Social psychologists borrowed the concept of skill from researchers interested in such things as performance in the work place, typing and the operation of automated plants. Social behaviour was, thus, seen to be a skill and could be treated as such – it could be decomposed into specific parts, it could be trained, shaped and improved. Indeed, Argyle [1978] noted: 'The model is simply this: that the sequence of individual behaviour which occurs during social interaction can usefully be looked at as a kind of motor skill. By motor skills are meant such things as cycling, skating, driving a car, playing the piano, typing, sending and receiving morse, performing industrial tasks, playing tennis and other games... Social interaction has many resemblances to other motor skills: the point of our suggestion is to pursue the basic psychological similarities in more detail, to see if the same processes operate' [pp. 59–60]. In pursuing this analogy between motor and social skills, Argyle [1978] simply borrowed a simple *motor skills model* (fig. 1) and adapted it to his purposes: 'I want to suggest that there is a useful analogy between motor skills like riding a bicycle, and social skills, like making friends, conducting conversations, and interviewing. In each case, the performer seeks certain goals, makes skilled moves which are intended to further them, observes what effect he is having, and takes corrective action as a result of feedback' [p. 63].

Problems with the adoption of the model will be discussed later, as will an emphasis on motor skills in early formulations which was subsequently dropped.

The history of SST in America was more rooted in clinical than occupational and social psychology [Furnham, 1985]. It stemmed originally out of the work of practising behaviour therapists who stressed social competence and assertiveness and the development of positive, pro-social behaviour [Phillips, 1985]. This approach is perhaps best summarized by Libet and Lewinson [1973], who provided a definition of social skills as: 'The complex ability both to emit behaviours which are positively or negatively reinforced and not to emit behaviours that are punished or extinguished by others' [p. 304]. A great deal of American SST remains the application of standard behaviourist therapies to social behavioural problems, many of which involve motor skills. Precisely because early behaviourists were more interested in observable behaviour, compared to cognition, there has always been an emphasis on motor behaviour, particularly nonverbal cues.

Despite the fact that the history of SST in Europe and North America is closely linked with an interest in movement, motor skills and nonverbal behaviour, various interesting developments have occurred, which will be discussed. However, it is first necessary to consider the theoretical basis of SST.

Theory or Theories

SST has been accused of being theoretically barren, methodologically weak and therapeutically ineffective. Whereas there is probably sufficient evidence to suggest that the latter two criticisms are false, it is highly likely that the former theoretical criticism is, indeed, true.

Before offering some general criticisms of the state of theory in SST it is important to note that some observers have complained that a unified, coherent or consistent theory does not exist; others that there are mutually competing or exclusive theories; still others that the theories that exist are weak or inadequate, and finally some argue that though there are adequate theories, practitioners ignore them [Stravinski, 1978; Yardley, 1979; Potter, 1982].

Clearly there are different approaches to SST because they have grown out of different branches of practice from micro-teaching to psychopathology, each with a different theoretical, practical, indeed epistemological base. Ellis and Whittington [1981] have suggested that there are four basic approaches to human learning which are reflected in the various SST programmes that exist:

(A) *Conditioning*: This is clearly the application of behaviourist theory and therapy to social behaviour, which might include verbal behaviour, gross motor behaviour or the minutiae of nonverbal behaviour. Through operant or classical conditioning the trainer seeks to shape social behaviour to some socially desirable and accepted norm. 'It should be noted at this point, however, that many of the necessary characteristics of the SST as a procedure for skill acquisition can be traced back to the conditioning paradigm. Thus, it is basic to SST that skills can be operationalized in terms of observable behaviour, that skills reduced to sub-skills are more easily acquired (and can be reconstituted by the trainee) and that reward (or at least association of appropriate response with pleasant consequences) is an important aspect of training' [p. 23]. As one may expect, because motor behaviour is more observable than cognitions, conditioning has been particularly successfully applied to nonverbal behaviour, such as eye gaze, gross body movements, smiling and gestures. It is probably true to say that this theoretical and consequential therapeutic approach has been more widely used in mental health settings than elsewhere, particularly in North America.

(B) *Cybernetic*: The critical aspect of this feedback approach includes an emphasis on the planned control of behaviour and the modification of cognitive strategies or tactical plans in the light of environmental feedback or knowledge of the consequences of action. This model is strictly based on a cognitive view of learning which explains skills' acquisition and maintenance in terms of unobservable internal events which can, and must, be inferred from external events. This approach differs from the previous one because it admits (indeed, finds essential) internal events; it accepts negative (as well as positive) feedback as being useful, and because feedback is thought to be intrinsically motivating. This approach is without doubt one of the most popular in the area because it stresses both the importance of cognitive variables like goals, scripts and plans *and* emphasizes the importance of feedback from others as a function of the behaviour itself.

(C) *Experimental*: This approach draws on such techniques as role play, psychodrama, T groups and experimental groups, and insists that in order to learn, people need to be exposed to an appropriate range of problem situations. People who are inadequate or unskilled are assumed to have not experienced enough, or any, of the situations that would allow them to learn. There is a strong idiographic streak in this approach which insists on wide individual differences and uniqueness, such that each person has to learn his/her particular solutions to everyday problems. Thus it is not assumed that any form of conditioning or feedback will help an individual, but rather that he or she has to 'work out' the appropriate skills for him- or herself. The popularity of this approach, however, is not great.

(D) *Teleological*: 'In the teleological paradigm it is assumed that analysis of, and subsequent commitment to, ends automatically generate effective means, and, furthermore, that explicit concern with means might inhibit creative and effective pursuit of ends. Thus a trainee would be encouraged to consider at length the purpose and patterns of effective interaction in his domestic, social or professional setting, but would be left to improvise his own technology of behaviour change to bring about improvement' [Ellis and Whittington, p. 26]. The training that follows from this approach is at one extreme, entirely theoretical in that trainer and trainee discuss possible behaviours in hypothetic situations. Again, the SST that follows from this approach is more armchair or couch-based than that found in the conditioning or cybernetic paradigm.

Clearly, the methodology one uses to investigate or experiment with social skills is a function of the approach one takes. Hence, researchers following the conditioning or cybernetic paradigm are likely to use empirical methods while those following the experimental or teleological models are likely to find an analytic or intuitive paradigm more appropriate.

Because of the diversity of approaches it is difficult to offer an all-encompassing critique of social skill theory. Nevertheless, some attempt will be made for four reasons: Firstly, the criticisms highlight differences between the various approaches. Secondly, because theory is the foundation of methodology and therapy it is hoped that increasing theoretical sophistication would lead to improvements in the research and practice of SST. Thirdly, by highlighting the major areas of concern a more programmatic research pattern into a highly diversified area may be encouraged. Finally, the criticisms may reveal the role of movement skills in SST more clearly.

Problems and Criticisms

Theoretical critiques of SST have revolved around numerous issues including the appropriateness and usefulness of *the* social skills model proposed by Argyle and Kendon [1967], and the definition of social skill. Although the social skills model was very roughly adapted from a perceptual and motor skill model, it has been extensively quoted by Argyle [Argyle, 1978, 1979; Trower et al. 1978] and others [Griffiths, 1980; Beattie, 1980] and has been described as a useful heuristic [Robinson, 1974]. For Argyle [1979]: 'This model has been heuristically very useful in drawing attention to the importance of feedback, and hence to gaze; it also suggests a number of different ways in which social performance can fail, and suggests the training procedures that may be effective through analogy with motor skills training' [p. 139]. It should be pointed out that although the section is specific to the cybernetic model proposed by Argyle and his colleagues, many, if not all, of the criticisms apply to the other models/theories as well.

In all fairness, it should be pointed out that Argyle [Argyle and Kendon, 1967; Argyle, 1979] has always been aware of the limitations of applying a model taken from perceptual and motor skills (man-machine interaction) and applying it to social behaviour. Hence special features of *social skill* have been pointed out which are not obviously present in manual skills such as the independent performance of the other person, the importance of taking the role of the other, strategies of self-presentation, the importance of rewarding-ness, the rules of social behaviour and the sequence of social events. Never-theless, the often repeated model shows no diagrammatic changes in order to modify it to be more appropriate for social behaviour.

Social Norms

Curiously the original model does not include any explicit reference to knowledge of social conventions, rules or, norms. In other words, if social and motor skills are situation and culture specific it is crucial that a person knows the social norms, as these dictate the appropriateness of behaviour. Trower [1980] has argued that social behaviour norms must be known to trainer and trainee before skills training can be effective – yet the model has no component of social knowledge. One important consequence of this omission is that the skills literature is highly culture specific [Furnham, 1979]. For instance, various researchers have shown that assertiveness is not always an indication of skill in other cultures. Humility, subservience and tolerance are valued above assertiveness in many other cultures, especially for women. Furthermore, lack of assertiveness is not necessarily a sign of inadequacy, though in instances it may be. More recently, Furnham and Bochner [1982], in an empirical analysis of culture shock, have suggested a social skills approach to culture learning. They argue that sojourners in a foreign culture who experience difficulty do so not because of intrapsychic conflicts but more simply because they do not know the skills of the host culture, or the norms of behaviour in it. Consequently, remedial action should not involve resolving unconscious conflicts, giving reassurance, systematic desensitiza-tion, or any similar technique. Rather help with culture shock involves imparting the appropriate knowledge about social norms and thence the skills, which may be achieved by using standard social skills' methods, such as instruction, modelling, role-playing, video-feedback and homework [Argyle, 1979]. In other words, a knowledge of social etiquette appropriate to one's milieu is an essential component in SST, yet neglected in models of SST.

Similarly, Welford [1981] has suggested that as different occupational classes are likely to be associated with different life-styles, interests, concerns and values, there are likely to be social class differences in social skills. These differences may lead to misunderstanding and misinterpretation, but if people from different classes are aware of the relevant differences in social norms and practices, they should have no difficulty in communicating with members from another social class.

Emotion

Many of the SST models neglected emotion which is, however, a central component in skill deficit – indeed skills deficit is often measured in terms of social anxiety [Watson and Friend, 1968]. Furthermore, the recognition of emotions in others is also considered an extremely important aspect of social skill [Argyle, 1978]. It is well known in human experimental psychology that heightened emotional arousal often leads to a reduction in performance. The model neglects an affective component which could affect other components of skill such as goals, perception and performance. The Yerkes-Dodson principle [Yerkes and Dodson, 1908] illustrates very well how it is possible to be overmotivated, creating a deleterious effect on performance. Extreme emotions of fear, anger or disgust are likely to disrupt social behaviour so causing the breakdown of social and motor skill. As a consequence, some researchers have maintained that many people do not need SST, but some form of desensitization because it is not that they lack skills but that their high anxiety levels prevent them from exercising those skilled behaviours. Yet many SST advocates would argue that anxiety is a function of lack of skills and hence the development of skills will, of necessity, reduce anxiety. However, very little work has been done attempting to ascertain the qualitative or quantitative effects of different emotions on social skills. This neglect may be due to the lack of emphasis on affect in the original model.

Perception

Another important criticism of the social skills' model is that three related, yet specific, types of social perception have been confounded and remain undistinguished in the model. That is, one may distinguish between person perception, self-monitoring and meta-perception [Pendleton and Furnham,

1980]. There is substantial literature on person perception, the perception of others [Cook, 1978], self-monitoring, the perception of oneself in social inter-action [Snyder, 1974], and meta-perception, the perception of others' percep-tion [Laing et al., 1966], which indicates that each process is important and unique in social interaction yet in social skills' literature these are often col-lapsed under the single process of social perception. Perhaps the most inter-esting and useful type of social perception to investigate from a therapeutic point of view is that of self-monitoring (or self-perception) which is a process concerned with self-presentation or impression management. Furnham and Capon [1983] have demonstrated that self-monitoring is an important com-ponent of social skills and that one should distinguish between perceptual sensitivity and behavioural flexibility in the self-monitoring process. That is, an individual may be able to perceive sensitively or monitor what behaviour is required and the impression that he/she is making, but be quite unable to modify or change that behaviour as he/she does not possess the relevant behavioural component of the social skill. People often perceive the need for assertiveness but are unable to behave in the appropriate fashion [Furnham and Henderson, 1981]. To use Goffman's [1959] and Snyder's [1974] 'life as theatre' analogy, both critics and actors may be high perceptual self-moni-tors but only the latter is able to act on his/her perception. The use of video cameras and role-play suggests the importance of self-monitoring in SST.

Unless the various types of perception are distinguished in the social skills' model, it is not clear whether social skills' perceptual deficits are due to inaccurate perception of others, faulty self-monitoring or incorrect meta-perceptions.

The Interactive Nature of the Model

Paradoxically, although the social skills' model is a model of social interaction, it is not itself interactive as there have been problems in specify-ing a two-person model, though some exist. Pendleton and Furnham [1980] attempted an interactive model of social skill when looking at the medical consultation. In order to make the model interactive, it was assumed that the patient has similar problems in understanding the doctor as the doctor has in understanding the patient. Though this model too has its problems, it is a step in the right direction.

The Definition of Social Skills

There are also problems with the definition of social skills. These differ enormously ranging from social adequacy in heterosexual situations through assertiveness and attentiveness, to giving appropriate self-disclosure. Phillips [1978] found 18 different, but related, definitions of skill before formulating his own: 'The extent to which he or she can communicate with others in a manner that fulfils one's right, requirements, satisfactions or obligations to a reasonable degree without damaging the other person's similar rights, requirements, satisfactions or obligations, and hopefully shares these rights etc. with others in free open exchange' [p. 13]. In one of their many reviews, Van Hasselt et al. [1979] have attempted to define social skill and, in doing so, highlighted three main elements which are seen to be crucial: social skills are situation specific; they are determined primarily by the learned acquisition and appropriate display of verbal and nonverbal response components, and they should enable people to behave in such a way as not to hurt or harm others. A more succinct definition which has five main features and which draws heavily on the work of Argyle is that of Hargie et al. [1981]: 'Social skill is a set of goal-directed, inter-related social behaviours which can be learned and which are under the control of the individual' [p. 13]. Wallace et al. [1980] have maintained that there are four major elements in most definitions of social skills: the patient's internal state (feelings, attitudes, perceptions); the topography of the patient's behaviour (the rate and latency particularly of nonverbal behaviours); the interaction as reflected in the achievement of the patient's goals, and the outcome of the interaction as reflected in the attitudes, feelings, behaviours and goals of other participants. They argue that a socially skilled response is the end result of a chain of behaviours that began with accurate 'perception' on relevant interpersonal stimuli, moved to flexible processing of these stimuli to generate and evaluate possible response options from which the correct one was chosen, and ended with appropriate 'sending' of the chosen option.

Curran [1979] has suggested that the plural term skills, as opposed to skill, has been used to connote the complexity of the response classes and the different typologies subsumed under this term. Further skill is often used in preference to competence or adequacy because of its neutral connotation. Curran has often offered a conceptual definition of skill in terms of behavioural consequences and general stylistic appropriateness.

One reason why there is so little agreement on the definition of social skills stems from the fact that there are four rather different models of SST.

The Components of Social Skill

One of the problems of the heterogeneity of definitions and traditions in SST is that each writer makes a different list of skills that constitute social skills. Ellis and Whittington [1981] have referred to a 'compendium of skills' when reviewing the lists of skills necessary in various training courses. These lists vary considerably in length, generality, etc. Compare the skills highlighted by Trower et al. [1978] (Observation, Listening, Speaking, Meshing, Expressing attitudes, Social routines, Tactics and strategies, and Situation training) with those of Hargie et al. [1981] (Nonverbal communication, Reinforcement, Questioning, Reflecting, Set induction and closure, Explanation, Listening and Self-Disclosure). The type of items included appear to relate to the background of the writer – hence Trower's list has a clinical flavour and Hargie's an educational theme. The precise number of skills specified appears to be randomly determined. Even within some skill lists there are surprising incongruities.

Ellis and Whittington [1981], in attempt to conceptualize the different dimensions along which skills appear to vary, have noted four:

(1) *Inference*: Low inference skills are easily observable and recordable whereas high inference skills such as sincerity require inference to be made from behaviour.

(2) *Molecularity*: Molecular skills such as mutual eye gaze are irreducible elements of interaction, whereas molar skills such as empathy or giving explanations are an amalgam of more molecular skills.

(3) *Specificality*: Situation-specific skills are relevant and appropriate only in a limited range of situations, whereas generic skills are relevant in very many situations.

(4) *Interactiveness*: Some interactive skills explicitly require the person to mesh his behaviour with that of others, whereas this may also be done implicitly.

Hence, there does not seem to be much consensus on the list of skills, their prevalence, how they may be recognized, or how they relate one to another logically and sequentially. Clearly more conceptual work, as outlined by Ellis and Whittington [1981], is needed in this field. As Romano and Bellack [1981] have pointed out: 'There is little empirical support for the particular components typically assessed as indices of social skill. These diverse response elements have been selected for study on the basis of face validity and general examination of the literature on interpersonal communication rather than on objective analysis of the various molar skill categories. Therefore, they may not represent the behaviours that actually contribute to social competence... The need for a clearly defined and operationalised set of behavioural referents of social skill has been noted by a number of researchers. Not only is it vital that the behaviours comprising social skill be specified but their optimal combination and weighting across different situations must be determined as well' [p. 479].

Empirical work on the components of social skills has in fact begun [McDonald and Cohen, 1981], but considerably more needs to be done. Continuous ambiguity as to the definition or operationalization of social skill means that SST subsumes a huge variety of techniques, ranging from behaviour therapy to non-directive counselling, which have been directed at widely different behaviours.

As yet, however, there exists no agreed-upon definition of social skills. To some extent this should not cause concern as there also exists no agreed-upon definition of psychology itself. Yet the plethora of very different definitions, some very specific and others very general, some coming obviously from a behavioural tradition, others from a more psychotherapeutic tradition, mean that under the flag of social skills one finds a very heterogeneous flotilla. For Curran [1980] 'The major problem which we must face squarely in the years to come is the definitional question: What is social skill and how can we best delimit and measure its components?' [p. 348].

Movement Skills in SST

Because there is no agreed definition of what social skills are, a wide variety of skills have been identified. Depending on the theoretical approach of the researcher, the setting in which he or she is operating, and the particular client/patient population that is being trained, very different skills lists emerge.

Consider the following three examples. Spence [1981] reported a study on SST with institutionalized juvenile male offenders. In all, she used 13 behavioural measures (table I) and found the offenders, as opposed to a control group, were significantly different (by being less skilled) in terms of eye contact, head movement, amount spoken, fiddling movements and gross body movements. Compared with the controls, the offender group were rated by six independent and 'blind' judges significantly less favourable in terms of social skills performance, social anxiety and employability. Latency of response, eye contact and head movements were significantly correlated with all four major judgements.

A different list of skills was drawn up by Burgess et al. [1980], working with sex offenders. They divided their skills into three categories thus: (1) *Eye contact*: intermittent (not staring); looking at the other person's face,

Table I. Definition and interjudge reliability of diverse behavioural variables [reprinted from Spence, 1981, with permission]

Behaviour variable	Definition	Interobserver reliability
Gestures, no/min	movements of hands or arms that clearly serve to illustrate or emphasize certain aspects of the conversation	0.93***
Fiddling, s/min	small movements of hands which are unrelated to content of speech, e.g. facial picking, scratching, hair stroking	0.99***
Gross body movements, no/min	large movements of arms, legs, or total body, resulting in a definite change in body position which is unrelated to content of conversation	1.00**
Smiling, no/min	upward movements of sides of mouth and cheeks, with or without accompanying sounds of laughter	0.99***
Appropriate head movements, no/min	up/down or side/side movements of head in which movement exceeded a one-inch deflection and which relates to an agreement or disagreement with some aspect of conversation	0.95***
Eye contact, s/min	subject looks directly into eyes of the interviewer both during listening and speaking	0.99***
Dysfluencies, no/min of speech	meaningless noises, e.g. umm, er, ah, or irrelevant pauses exceeding 0.5 s duration made during speech	0.93***
Attention feedback responses, no/min	verbal responses made during listening role including acknowledgements, e.g. mm, yes, I see, and question feedback responses, e.g. oh? did you? really? One response was counted for any sequence of responses in each 5 s interval	0.89***
Amount spoken, s/min	all verbal utterances made during interview	0.80**
Interruptions, no/min	verbal initiations made by listener before interviewer completes utterance; excludes attention feedback responses which do not aim to take over speaker role	1.00***
Questions asked, no/min	verbal initiations made which request information from interviewer; excludes question feedback responses or requests for repetition of data	0.80**
Initiations, no/min	verbal statements which place person into speaker role other than questions, interruptions or responses to interviewer's questions	0.76**
Latency of response, s/response	time between interviewer's questions and subject's verbal response	0.98***

** $p < 0.01$, ***$p < 0.001$.

and responsive (showing attention). (2) *Voice control*: appropriately loud; clear, and modulated (avoid monotony). (3) *Body*: relaxed, with appropriate gestures; orientated towards the other person, and face not concealed, appropriate facial expression.

Again, a quite different list of skills served as the target for training in a study by Schinke et al. [1979], who were concerned with training staff from a social service agency in a natural setting. The eight skills that were the focus of their attention were: (1) *Eye contact*: length of time subjects looked at the confederate's eyes; rated for all vignettes. (2) *Smiles*: frequency of smiles during each vignette; rated for all vignettes. (3) *Positive affective responses*: frequency of statements indicating liking for confederate's responses, character traits or behaviour (e.g. 'I enjoy being with you'). (4) *Appreciation*: frequency of statements indicating gratitude for confederate's behaviour (e.g. 'Thank you for a nice evening'). (5) *No statements*: frequency of S use of 'no'. (6) *Compliance*: occurrence of S acquiescence to confederate's demands. (7) *Refusals*: frequency of statements indicating unwillingness to conform with confederate's suggestions or demands. (8) *Requests for new behaviour*: frequency of statements asking confederates to change behaviour. Viewed on a continuum, compliance was not resisting a confederate demand, refusal was active resistance, and request for new behaviour was active resistance plus a counterdemand.

What is apparent from these three different studies is that various quite different behaviours are targeted for skills training. It is possible to break these down into three different groups – verbal, vocal, nonverbal – of which the latter is concerned specifically with motor aspects. Verbal skills, as one may imagine, are concerned with the appropriateness of questions, answers and statements; the number and type of interruptions, initiations and responses; the absolute amount of time spent talking, etc. Vocal behaviours are more concerned with dysfluencies, the appropriateness of pitch, loudness, etc., and the amount of vocal feedback given to others. It is in the area of nonverbal behaviour that SST researchers are most concerned with movement skills.

There are probably many ways in which nonverbal movement skills could be classified, but the scheme outlined in table II may be a useful beginning. Of course, it may well be possible to treat molar movements, i.e. gesture on a molecular level and vice versa, namely treating molecular movements, i.e. smiling on a molar level of analysis. But it is probably true to say that head and facial features have nearly all been treated at the molecular level, while body movements have most frequently been treated at the molar

Table II. A classification of nonverbal movement skills

	Head	Body
Molar	nodding shaking	posture gesture proximity
Molecular	smiling gaze patterns eyebrow movements pupil dilation	fiddling leg/arm movements

level. There are probably good reasons for this – the face, particularly the eyes and mouth, are probably the richest source of nonverbal communication in the sense that very small movements have considerable significance, while body movements are frequently more gross and hence less culturally transmitted information.

What questions do social skills' trainers and researchers pose with respect to movement skills? A number are frequently asked:

(A) *What do the movements mean?* There are essentially two parts to this question. That is, is there a shared definition as to what certain movements mean? Do the movements have a psychological significance for the sender *and* receiver of the messages or are the results purely epiphenomenal?

The first question has considerably stimulated research, particularly with respect to motor behaviours such as gestures and head movements. In an extensive study of 20 key gestures (involving hand, head and arm movements) in 40 locations over Western Europe, Morris et al. [1979] attempted to understand the universality in the interpretation of gestures. They found that gestures had several major meanings and that the phenomenon of the multimessage gesture stems from the frequent, local selection of different symbolic pathways. They also found that many of the gestures extended their ranges across national and linguistic boundaries, but that some stopped abruptly, within a linguistic area. Some gestures showed an interesting colonial pattern, giving high scores in an old imperial power (i.e. Greece and Rome) and also in one of its ex-colonies, despite being absent or rare in the geographically intervening regions. Gestures then, which are quite deliberate nonverbal signals that frequently accompany speech, do have shared meanings but these meanings are historically, geographically and linguistically determined.

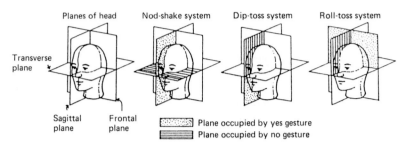

Fig. 2. Systems of affirmation and negation. [Reprinted from Collett, 1982, with permission.]

In a particularly interesting example, Collett [1982] has considered the meaning of head movements in three planes: frontal, sagittal and transverse. From this he has been able to detect three quite different and distinct codes for 'yes' and 'no' (fig. 2).

The most common is the 'nod-shake code' which involves a movement of the head up and down in the sagittal plane for 'yes', and a movement from side to side in the transverse plane for 'no'. Alternatively, the 'dip-toss code' has a downward movement of the head in the sagittal plane to signal 'yes' and an upward movement in the same plane to indicate 'no'. Finally, the 'roll-toss code' rolls the head across the shoulders in the frontal plane for 'yes', and an upward movement of the head in the sagittal plane for 'no'. As Collett [1982] points out, the codes select *different* tracts of the motor territory available to express signals; certain movements do not make a distinction with respect to initial direction of movement, while others do and that quite distinct kinemes for one culture or society may simply be allokinemes of the same kineme for another. It seems, therefore, that many ritualized gestures and movements do have meaning, but that these meanings differ from one region to another.

(B) *To what extent are senders vs. receivers aware of movements?* It often seems paradoxical that the nonverbal movements which are most dramatic and extensive (change in body posture) may be those of which either the sender or receiver is unaware. Argyle [1975] has suggested a number of possibilities for nonverbal communication (table III). Notice that two motor skills – spatial behaviour and body posture – are considered examples of behaviour where either the sender or the receiver of the message is unaware. Presumably one of the aims of social skills trainings is to make both parties aware of their own and others' movements *and* their meaning.

Table III. Awareness of movement amongst senders and receivers [Argyle, 1975]

Sender	Receiver	
Aware	aware	verbal communication, some gestures, e.g. pointing
Mostly unaware	mostly aware	most NVC
Unaware	unaware, but has an effect	pupil dilation, gaze shifts and other small nonverbal signals
Aware	unaware	sender is trained in the use of e.g. spatial behaviour
Unaware	aware	receiver is trained in the interpretation of e.g. bodily posture

(C) *How easy are motor skills to train?* Many researchers interested in motor skills are interested in fine, highly skilled behaviour that may be found in certain sports or activities like singing. The skills involved are manifold, and considerable practice is necessary. As regards the motor skills component of social skills the problem is far less complicated. The number and type of movements that are required are both relatively limited and simple. For instance, a person could be taught to send and receive information through gesture and body posture comparatively easily. Indeed, a lot of training does not go into the development of specific skills but into attempts to relax subjects sufficiently to prevent gauche, erratic movements or continually twitching and fidgeting, which is off-putting. In other words, many movements may be seen as displacement behaviour more than actual communication.

Motor behaviour, at least on the macro-level (changes in body posture) vs. micro-level (changes in eye contact patterns) is fairly easy to train and frequently inappropriate movements are seen as simply the consequences of anxiety rather than the absence of skill.

(D) *Are changes in motor behaviour more important than 'steady-state' positions?* Much of the work on motor behaviour within the SST paradigm has been to identify specific postures, gestures and spatial patterns, and to explore how to 'encode' interpersonal attitudes. However, because many movements carry relatively little information in themselves, it has been suggested that changes in movement, especially when in the interaction they occur is as, if not more, important than the movements themselves. The timing of movements, therefore, may convey more information than how or what is being moved.

There may be other questions that SST researchers and practitioners ask in this field, but it remains the case that motor skills are still relatively neglected.

Current Concerns and Future Interests

After a period of rapid expansion and application to numerous populations and settings, SST has gone through a period of critical evaluation and empirical assessment [Curran, 1979; Furnham, 1983; Trower, 1980]. Recently a number of 'Handbooks' [L'Abate and Milan, 1985; Hollin and Trower, 1986] and 'Critiques' have been published in the area [Trower, 1984; Ellis and Whittington, 1983].

Hollin and Trower [1986] have critically and succinctly offered a critique of SST and possible future developments. They divided this into three areas. There remain various *technical* issues, such as how to assess social skills (by questionnaire, role play, physiological measures); the most effective and efficient training method, and the persistent problem of the generalization of skills across time and situations. There also remains the issue of the abuse of SST, either by claiming any type of 'therapy' is SST, or else insufficient evaluative research being performed and numerous exaggerated and unsubstantial claims being made of it.

However, perhaps the most interesting developments are theoretical, and here can be detected considerable tension between two quite different developments. The *radical behaviour* position does not deny the role of cognitions and private experiences, but does not allow them to be considered as 'autonomous causes of behaviour'. Yet cognitions are treated as not publicly observable behaviours which can be trained. For instance, this approach allows for training in social perception (modelling and instruction as to which social cues should be attended to, and how they should be decoded); social cognition (increasing knowledge of response alternatives and the learning of social rules and conventions) and social performance (shaping up to new, overt, social behaviours). Opposed to this approach are *radical cognitivists* who set great store by the way people understand and process social phenomena. They sometimes distinguish between social *skills* – the various normative behaviours which a person needs in a repertoire, and social *skill* – the ability to put these into practice. Trower [1980] has argued that the former was widely practised and the latter sadly neglected. He advocates a new radical cognitivism which stresses the importance of social rules, the moral order of social behaviour and the construction of meaning. Apart from being strongly opposed to cybernetic or conditioning approaches, however, it is unclear how SST will proceed under the new order.

To a large extent, these two approaches are reactions to the 'cognitive revolution' that has overtaken SST, as with other areas. More and more emphasis was placed on the perception of social behaviour: Scripts and goals for action; lack of understanding of the rules of social behaviour; rather than on actual behaviour. Whereas this may be seen to be 'corrective' on the early too behavioural emphasis in earlier training, it is quite possible that the balance has swung too far.

Psychologists interested in SST have only been peripherally interested in the theoretical and methodological issues faced by action and motor skills theorists, such as whether the control of action is a cognitive process; whether motor learning is like regression; how anticipation is involved in movement production; whether muscles are like springs, and whether knowledge of results (feedback) is necessary for learning [Harvey, 1988].

However, there do appear to be some parallels. For instance, the tension between a cognitive versus a behaviourist approach may not be found with those interested in both social and motor skill. There also appears to be something of a gulf between those that apply social and motor skills theories in 'real-world settings' (i.e. mental hospitals, sports clinics) and those who do experimental work with, and speculate upon, those theories.

Areas of Application

SST has many possible applications including the area of sport and movement. By definition, SST is concerned with human interaction and the shaping of interpersonal behaviours relevant to social intercourse. It seems therefore particularly appropriate for highly social sports such as team sports as opposed to more individual sports. Three areas seem particularly important – the first concerns the effect of anxiety on skilled performance and the possibility of behaviouristic SST to reduce anxiety to optimal levels. Secondly where sports involve such things as deception, SST can be used to help people actually become more sensitive to the detection of deception in others but also learn to deceive others more successfully. Finally, because efficient and effective communication is so important in team sports it may be possible to train team members in a specific vocal or visual language that ideally serves their purposes while simultaneously being unknown to other teams.

Finally, motor scientists could learn both from the range of techniques used in SST but also in studying how movements are perceived. Because many movements carry specific psychological messages, it may be useful to consider not only the shaping of physical movement but the impression it carries to the perceiver of those movements.

Social skills trainers and researchers have by and large neglected the rich and developing literature in movement theory. Perhaps this book will help to encourage closer contact between movement and social skills trainers and researchers.

References

Argyle, M.: Bodily communication (Methuen, London 1975).

Argyle, M.: The psychology of interpersonal behaviour; 3rd ed. (Penguin, Harmondsworth 1978).

Argyle, M.: New developments in the analysis of social skills; in Wolfgang, Nonverbal behaviour: Applications and cross-cultural implication (Academic Press, New York 1979).

Argyle, M.; Bryant, B.; Trower, P.: Social skills training and psychotherapy: A comparative study. Psychol. Med. *4:* 435–444 (1974).

Argyle, M.; Kendon, A.: The experimental analysis of social performance. Adv. exp. soc. Psychol. *3:* 55–98 (1967).

Beattie, G.: The skilled art of conversational interaction; in Singleton, Spurgeon, Stammers, The analysis of social skills (Plenum, New York 1980).

Burgess, R.; Jewitt, R.; Sandham, J.; Hudson, B.: Working with sex offenders: A social skills training group. Br. J. soc. Work *10:* 133–142 (1980).

Cook, M.: The social skill model and interpersonal attraction; in Duck, Theory and practice in interpersonal attraction (Academic Press, London 1978).

Collett, P.: Meetings and misunderstandings; in Bochner, Cultures in contact (Pergamon, Oxford 1982).

Curran, J.: Pandora's box reopened? The assessment of social skills. J. behav. Assess. *1:* 55–71 (1979).

Ellis, R.; Whittington, D.: A guide to social skills training (Croom Helm, London 1981).

Ellis, R.; Whittington, D.: New directions in social skill training (Croom Helm, London 1982).

Furnham, A.: Assertiveness in three cultures: Multidimensionality and cultural differences. J. clin. Psychol. *35:* 522–527 (1979).

Furnham, A.: Research in social skills training: A critique; in Ellis, Whittington, New directions in social skills training (Croom Helm, London 1983).

Furnham, A.: Social skills training: A European Perspective; in L'Abate, Milan, Handbook of social skills training and research, pp. 555–580 (Wiley, New York 1985).

Furnham, A.: Social skills training with adolescents and young adults; in Hollin, Trower, Handbook of social skills training, pp. 33–57 (Pergamon, Oxford 1986).

Furnham, A.; Bochner, S.: Social difficulty in a foreign culture: An empirical analysis of culture shock; in Bochner, Culture in contact: Studies in cross-cultural interaction, (Pergamon, Oxford 1982).

Furnham, A.; Capon, M.: Social skills and self-monitoring processes. Personal. Individ. Diff. *4:* 171–178 (1983).

Furnham, A.; Henderson, M.: Sex differences in self-reported assertiveness in Britain. Br. J. clin. Psychol. *20:* 50–62 (1981).

Goffman, E.: The presentation of self in everyday life (Edinburgh University Press, Edinburgh 1959).

Gresham, F.: Validity of social skills measures of assessing social skills in low status children. Dev. Psychol. *17:* 390–398 (1981).

Griffiths, R.: Social skills and psychological disorder; in Singleton, Spurgeon, Stammers, The analysis of social skills (Plenum, New York 1980).

Hargie, O.; Saunders, C.; Dickson, D.: Social skills in interpersonal communication (Croom Helm, London 1981).

Harvey, N.: The psychology of action: Current controversies; in Claxton, New horizons in cognition (Routledge & Kegan Paul, London 1988).

Hollin, C.; Trower, P.: Handbook of social skills training, vol. I + II (Pergamon, Oxford 1986).

L'Abate, L.; Milan, M.: Handbook of social skills training and research (Wiley, New York 1985).

Laing, R.; Phillipson, H.; Lee, A.: Interpersonal perception (Tavistock, London 1966).

Libet, J.; Lewinson, P.: Concept of social skills with special reference to the behaviour of depressed persons. J. consult. clin. Psychol. *40:* 304–312 (1973).

McDonald, M.; Cohen, J.: Trees in the forest: Some components of social skills. J. clin. Psychol. *37:* 342–347 (1981).

Morris, D.; Collett, P.; Marsh, P.; O'Shaughnessy, M.: Gestures: The origin and distribution (Cape, London 1979).

Oei, T.; Jackson, P.: Long-term effects of group and individual social skills training with alcoholics. Addict. Behav. *5:* 129–136 (1980).

Pendleton, D.; Furnham, A.: Skills: A paradigm for applied social psychological research; in Singleton, Spurgeon, Stammers, The analysis of social skill (Plenum, New York 1980).

Phillips, E.: The social skills bases of psychopathology (Grune & Stratton, London 1978).

Phillips, E.: Social skills: History and prospect; in L'Abate, Milan, Handbook of social skills training and research, pp. 3–21 (Wiley, New York 1985).

Potter, J.: 'Nothing as practical as good theory...'. The problematic application of social psychology; in Stringer, Confronting social issues: Applications of social psychology (Academic Press, London 1982).

Robinson, W.: Language and social behaviour (Penguin, Harmondsworth 1974).

Romano, J.; Bellack, A.: Social validation of a component model of assertive behaviour. J. consult. clin. Psychol. *48:* 478–490 (1981).

Schinke, S.; Gilchrist, L.; Smith, T.; Wong, S.: Group interpersonal skills training in a natural setting: An experimental study. Behav. Res. Ther. *17:* 149–154 (1979).

Snyder, M.: The self-monitoring of expressive behaviour. J. Pers. soc. Psychol. *30:* 226–237 (1974).

Spence, S.: Differences in social skills performance between institutionalized juvenile male offenders and a comparable group of boys without offence records. Br. J. clin. Psychol. *20:* 163–172 (1981).

Spence, S.; Marzillier, J.: Social skills training with adolescent male offenders. II. Short-term, long-term and generalized effects. Behav. Res. Ther. *19:* 349–368 (1981).

Stravinski, A.: The 'Emperor's Clothes' revealed or social skills vs. research skills. Behav. Psychother. *6:* 91–96 (1978).

Trower, P.: Situational analysis of the components and processes of behaviour of socially skilled and unskilled patients. J. consult. clin. Psychol. *48:* 327–339 (1980).

Trower, P.; Bryant, B.; Argyle, M.: Social skills and mental health (Methuen, London 1978).

Van Hasselt, V.; Hersen, M.; Whitehill, M.; Bellack, A.: Social skills assessment and training for children. Behav. Res. Ther. *17:* 413–437 (1979).

Wallace, C.; Nelson, C.; Liberman, R.; Aitchinson, R.; Lukoff, D.; Elder, J.; Ferris, C.: A review and critique of social skills training with schizophrenic patients. Schizophrenia Bull. *6:* 42–65 (1980).

Watson, D.; Friend, R.: Measurement of social-evaluative anxiety. J. consult. clin. Psychol. *33:* 448–457 (1968).

Welford, A.: Social skills and social class. Psychol. Rep. *48:* 847–852 (1981).

Yardley, K.: Social skills training: A critique. Br. J. med. Psychol. *52:* 55–62 (1979).

Yerkes, R.; Dodson, J.: The relation of strength of stimulus to rapidity of habit formulation. J. comp. neurol. Psychol. *18:* 459–491 (1908).

Adrian Furnham, DPhil, Department of Psychology, University College London, 26 Bedford Way, London WC1H OAP (UK)

Subject Index